KEYS TO MEDICAL ASSISTING
A Pocket Guide

Jahangir Moini, M.D., M.P.H.
Professor of Science and Health,
Eastern Florida State College

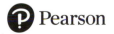 Pearson   330 Hudson Street, NY NY 10013

Vice President, Health Science and TED: Julie Levin Alexander
Director, Portfolio Management: Marlene McHugh Pratt
Editor in Chief: Ashley Dodge
Portfolio Management Assistant: Emily Edling
Associate Sponsoring Editor: Zoya Zaman
Product Marketing Manager: Rachele Strober
Field Marketing Manager: Brittany Hammond
Vice President, Digital Studio and Content Production Paul DeLuca
Director, Digital Studio and Content Production: Brian Hyland

Managing Producer: Jennifer Sargunar
Content Producer (Team Lead): Faraz Sharique Ali
Content Producer: Neha Sharma
Senior Manager, Global Rights and Permissions: Tanvi Bhatia
Operations Specialist: Maura Zaldivar-Garcia
Cover Design: Cenveo Publisher Services
Cover Photo: Jahangir Moini
Full-Service Management and Composition: iEnergizer Aptara®, Ltd.
Printer/Binder: LSC Communications, Inc.
Cover Printer: Phoenix Color
Text Font: 9.75/10.75, Times LT Pro

Library of Congress Cataloging-in-Publication Data
Names: Moini, Jahangir, 1942- author.
Title: Keys to medical assisting : pocket guide / Jahangir Moini, M.D., M.P.H.
Description: Second edition. | Hoboken : Pearson, [2018] | Includes bibliographical references and index.
Identifiers: LCCN 2018015187 | ISBN 9780134868295 | ISBN 0134868293
Subjects: LCSH: Medical assistants—Handbooks, manuals, etc. | Medical offices—Management—Handbooks, manuals, etc.
Classification: LCC R728.8 .M652 2018 | DDC 610.73/7—dc23 LC record available at https://lccn.loc.gov/2018015187

1 18

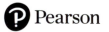

ISBN-13: 978-0-13-486829-5
ISBN-10:   0-13-486829-3

*This book is dedicated to the memory of my Mother;
to my wife, Hengameh; to my daughters, Mahkameh
and Morvarid; and to my granddaughters, Laila Jade
and Anabelle Jasmine Mabry*

CONTENTS

Keys to Medical Assisting: A Pocket Guide, Second Edition is designed to be an easy-to-use reference for both students and practicing medical assistants in the healthcare field. Small enough to fit in your pocket, this book will come in handy whether in the externship or on the job.

The chapters flow from the more basic information that is required in this field to the more complex knowledge areas that must also be attained. For further ease of use, the chapters are divided into five sections: *Administrative Medical Assisting*, *Office Equipment and Financial Management*, *Clinical Medical Assisting*, *Laboratory Procedures*, and *Basic Pharmacology and Administration of Medications*.

The book's appendices, designed for quick reference, focus on a variety of unique topics and contain readily understandable terms and concepts.

This guide will provide students and professionals more confidence as they will have a ready-reference guide in their pocket.

New to This Edition

1. Chapter 1 has been retitled to "Introduction and General Office Duties"
2. Chapter 2 is a new chapter, entitled "Using Computers in the Office"
3. Chapter 6 has been retitled to "Forms of Communication"
4. Chapter 7 has been retitled to "Managing Supplies and Banking"
5. Chapter 9 has been retitled to "Diagnostic and Procedural Coding"

6. Chapter 15 has been retitled to "Diagnostic Phlebotomy and Hematology"

7. Chapter 19 has been retitled to "Principles of Pharmacology"

8. Appendix B has been retitled to "Common Medical Terms and Misspelled Terms"

9. Appendix E has been retitled to "MyPlate Dietary Guidelines"

10. Appendix F has been retitled to "Nutrition (Vitamins and Minerals)"

11. Appendix G has been retitled to "CMA, RMA, CCMA, and NCMA Examinations"

For all of these updates, a lot of new information has been added.

- Some of the figures and illustrations have been moved from the book to the student resources website (SRS).
- There are also some new illustrations that have been added.
- All drugs listed in the book have been updated.
- All immunization schedules and their footnotes, for children and adults, have been updated.

Student Supplement

Some of the appendices, figures, and tables referred in the book are appearing on the student resources website (SRS) www.pearsonhighered.com/healthprofessionsresources
Click on view all resources and select Medical Assisting from the choice of disciplines. Find this book and you will find the respective appendices, figures, and tables.

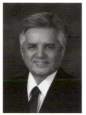

Dr. Jahangir Moini

Dr. Jahangir Moini was an assistant professor at Tehran University School of Medicine for 9 years, teaching medical and allied health students. Dr. Moini was a professor and former director (for 15 years) of allied health programs at Everest University. He reestablished the Medical Assisting Program, in 1990, at Everest University's Melbourne campus. He also established several other new allied health programs for Everest University.

From 2000 to 2007, Dr. Moini was a physician liaison of the Florida Society of Medical Assistants. He has been a marketing strategy team member of the American Association of Medical Assistants (AAMA) and president of the Brevard County chapter of the AAMA. Since 1999, Dr. Moini has been a published author of 20 allied health books. Currently, he is a professor of science and health at Eastern Florida State College.

ACKNOWLEDGMENTS

This pocket guide is the culmination of the efforts of many people, including my medical assisting students of many years, who inspired me to write it. On the publishing and production side at Pearson, I would like to thank Julie Levin Alexander, Vice President/Publisher; Marlene Pratt, Editorial Director; and Neha Sharma, Content Producer.

My special thanks go to Greg Vadimsky, who has been beside me from the initiation of the proposal and the project until the end.

I would also like to thank the following reviewers for pushing me to create the best pocket guide I could:

Ron Maly, MA, RMA (AMT), CPhT (PTCB)
CHI/St. Elizabeth Hospital
Lincoln, Nebraska

Paula D. Silver, Pharm D
ECPI University
Newport News, Virginia

Lisa Rosenau, ASMA, BsHS, MsED
Keiser University
Fort Lauderdale, Florida

Shelina Macarthur, MA
Ultimate Medical Academy
Clearwater, Florida

Peter F. Andrus, MD
Albany Medical College
Albany, New York

Jacqueline G. McRae-Mitchell, MEd., CMA-AAMA,
AHI (AMT)
South College
Knoxville, Tennessee

Karmle L Conrad, MHA, CPC, CMA, RPT
Health Care Consultant
Sandwich, Massachusetts

SECTION I
Administrative Medical Assisting

CHAPTER 1
Introduction and General Office Duties

The duties of medical assistants include administrative, clinical, and laboratory work. Administrative duties of medical assistants are as important as clinical duties. Each medical practice may require different, specific tasks to be done each day.

MEDICAL ASSISTING ORGANIZATIONS

There are several professional organizations related to medical assisting. These include the American Association of Medical Assistants (AAMA), American Medical Technologists (AMT), the National Healthcareer Association (NHA), and the National Center for Competency Testing (NCCT). Each of these organizations offers a different medical assisting certification (see Table 1-1).

DUTIES OF THE RECEPTIONIST

A receptionist's duties and responsibilities include the following:

- Opening and closing the office
- Greeting patients as they arrive
- Signing in patients
- Helping new patients fill out paperwork
- Answering patients' questions
- Assisting patients in filling out paperwork
- Collecting records of patients

Table 1-1 *Medical Assisting Certifications*

Organization	Credential	Fees	Notes
American Association of Medical Assistants (AAMA) http://www.aama-ntl.org/cma-aama-exam 800-228-2262	CMA (5 years)	$125 for recent graduates and members, $250 for others	Not-for-profit. Annual fees $25 to $40 for students, up to $107 for others, all based on state.
American Medical Technologists (AMT) https://www.americanmedtech.org 847-823-5169	RMA (3 years)	$120	Not-for-profit. Annual fees $50.
National Healthcareer Association (NHA) http://www.nhanow.com/certifications/clinical-medical-assistant 800-499-9092	CCMA (2 years)	$149	For-profit.
National Center for Competency Testing (NCCT) https://www.ncctinc.com/certifications/ma.aspx 800-875-4404	NCMA (1 year)	$90 for recent graduates, $135 for others	For-profit.

Category	Topics Covered
General (or Basic)	Medical terminology Anatomy and physiology Behavioral science; psychology Medical law and ethics
Administrative	Oral and written communication Records management Insurance and coding Computers and office machines Bookkeeping, collections, and credit Law and ethics
Clinical	Examination room techniques and procedures Laboratory techniques and procedures Pharmacology and medication administration Emergency procedures Specimen collection Diagnostic tests

Note: All of these examinations are basically the same, covering the topics listed above. The CCMA lists "Basic, Administrative, and Clinical," while the CMA and RMA exams list "General, Administrative, and Clinical." The NCMA has 13 content categories, but these cover the same basic required knowledge as the other exams.

- Writing chart slips
- Updating patient demographics
- Calling for patient insurance verification
- Answering incoming calls
- Handling patients' complaints
- Making sure that the reception area is safe and clean
- Scheduling return appointments
- Documenting patient no-shows

Steps for Opening the Office

Medical assistants or receptionists must open the office 15–30 minutes before the start of office hours. When the office opens, the following procedures are required:

- Turning on the lights
- Disengaging the alarm system
- Starting up the computers
- Checking the heating or air-conditioning
- Observing the reception area for safety hazards, such as
  - Carpeting that is easy to clean
  - Frayed electrical cords
  - Slippery floors
  - Torn carpeting
- Placing a warning sign near a potential safety hazards
- Checking magazines and recycling any that are damaged or outdated
- Checking the level of cleanliness as kept up by housekeeping services
- Taking calls from the answering machine or answering service
- Checking the late-night pickup specimen boxes to ensure that all items were taken

- Printing a list of the patients scheduled and distributing it to the physician(s)
- Gathering any laboratory test information that is missing from a patient's record
- Immediately reporting the hazard
- Unlocking file rooms or cabinets
- Unlocking the outer office door

Registration Information

The registration of a new patient may require a registration form, a private area to conduct the registration, a pen, a clipboard, and other clerical supplies. The information required to register a patient's first visit may include the following:

- Full name
- Birth date
- Spouse's name
- Home address and telephone number
- Social security number, driver's license number, or other identification number
- Occupation and the name, address, and phone number of their employer
- Referring physician
- Name and address of the person, if other than the patient, who is responsible for payment
- Method of payment
- Primary health insurance information

  - Type of coverage
  - Group policy number
  - Subscriber number
  - Assignment of benefits

Collating Medical Records

Medical assistants must prepare medical records for review by the physician. The following steps are required:

- Typing a list of all patients and printing the patients' appointment schedule
- Pulling the medical records of scheduled patients
- Reviewing the patients' last appointment
- Arranging the charts sequentially according to appointment time
- Making notes of any results that are received, including
  - Laboratory test results
  - X-ray results
  - Consultation notes
- Putting all information that is received onto the chart
- Placing the charts in the appropriate examination room

Answering the Telephone

Callers often receive their first impression of the medical office through a phone call. When answering the phone, be sure to

- Smile
- Use the office greeting
- Watch your speech patterns, including
  - Clarity
  - Enunciation
  - Inflection
  - Pitch
- Identify the caller by name

Key Focus: The medical assistant must always avoid responding negatively to angry callers and should attempt to help with the root of the caller's real problem.

> **Key Focus:** The medical assistant must hold the telephone's mouthpiece about 1 inch from the mouth when speaking.

On-Hold Callers

One of the most sensitive issues relating to telephone courtesy is the use of the "hold" function. It is important to allow a second caller time to respond before placing him or her on hold. If a second call is an emergency, you must take care of the caller before returning to an original call. The following should be avoided when placing a caller on hold:

- Switching the caller to "hold" before he or she states the reason for the call
- Placing several callers on hold at the same time
- Going back to the "hold" call and asking "Who are you waiting for?"
- Cutting off calls by careless use of the hold button
- Leaving a caller "on hold" for several minutes without checking back
- Playing loud music on the telephone line while a patient is "on hold"
- Stating rudely to "hold" or "hold please" without giving any explanation

Taking Messages

When taking a message, make sure that correct and relevant information is retrieved. Message forms or pads with carbon paper must be kept permanently near the phone. They must contain the following information about the call and the caller:

- Full name and telephone number
- Time and date

- Complete message as received
- Initials of the person taking the message

Incoming Calls and Triage

Patients may call for the following reasons:

- Appointment requests
- Insurance and billing questions
- Questions about fees
- Requests for office hours and directions
- Questions about laboratory test results
- Prescription refills
- Requests for referrals
- Follow-up calls
- To speak with the physician

If you receive calls from patients, the following information must be requested:

- Name
- Telephone number
- Time and date of the call
- The patient's physician, if in a multi-physician practice
- Insurance information
- Nature of the problem

Nonpatient Calls

Other incoming calls may include the following:

- Calls from sales representatives
- General office business calls
- Personal calls for the physician
- Other physicians' calls
- Calls from a pharmacy, requiring information from the physician
- Reports from hospitals
- Prank calls

Key Focus: Know your office policy and your physician's preferences for handling nonpatient calls.

Emergency Calls

Generally, medical assistants may be faced with the following types of emergency calls:

- Allergic reaction to drugs
- Drug overdose
- Heart attack
- Loss of consciousness
- Severe bleeding
- Broken bones
- Asthma attack
- Premature labor
- Suicide attempts
- Gunshot wounds
- Stabbing wounds
- Injury of the eyes
- High fever

Clinical Responsibilities

The medical assistant also has clinical responsibilities, which are as follows:

- Assisting the physician during examinations
- Administering vaccines and injections
- Performing phlebotomy
- Performing ECGs
- Performing CPR
- Preparing patients for examinations
- Assisting with minor surgery
- Taking vital signs and medical history

General Office Duties

- Sterilizing medical instruments
- Teaching patients
- Following Occupational Safety and Health Administration (OSHA) guidelines

Laboratory duties include the following:
- Meeting OSHA guidelines
- Performing Clinical Laboratory Improvement Amendment (CLIA) procedures
- Collecting, preparing, and transmitting laboratory specimens
- Arranging for laboratory services

Chapter 2
Using Computers in the Office

Today's medical offices utilize computers, software, and various types of administrative equipment on a daily basis. Medical assistants must know how to operate, maintain, troubleshoot, and sometimes purchase or lease this equipment. Computers are a regular part of the following:

- Billing patients
- Submitting claims
- Bank deposits
- Payroll
- Communications, especially e-mail

Other equipment used in the medical office includes

- Copiers
- Scanners
- Calculators
- Paper shredders
- Fax machines

COMPUTERS

Computers are used in the medical office, commonly as part of a *network*. This is a system linking computers together. One computer acts as a *server*, which stores the information shared on the network. An example of this stored information is the office's *database management system*. Types of computers include

- Desktop—fits on a desk or other flat surface; usually has a *tower case* placed on the floor

- Laptop and notebook—only about the size of a magazine, these are very light computers, operating on batteries or electrical outlet power; they are easy to move to different areas of the office
- Tablet PC and subnotebook—small mobile computers with touch screens, operated with a stylus, digital pen, or the user's finger (instead of a keyboard or mouse)
- Personal digital assistant (PDA)—less common today than in previous years, PDAs were primarily used to look up reference information, and to enter information into patient's charts

Various types of computers are shown in Figure 2-1.

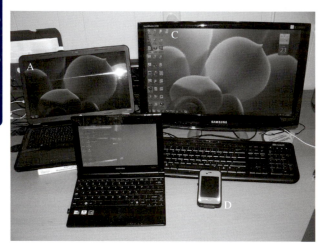

Figure 2-1 *Types of computers: (A) laptop, (B) notebook, (C) desktop, and (D) smartphone.*

Key Focus: Medical office computers usually have *encryption software* installed to protect private health information. Other types of security software, including *passwords*, are used to ensure that all computer users have permission to access specific information.

Frequently used computer terms are listed in Table 2-1.

Table 2-1 *Frequently Used Computer Terms*

Term	Definition
backup	A copy of work or software batch data stored for processing at periodic intervals
batch	Data stored for processing at periodic intervals
boot	To start up a computer
catalog	List of all files stored on a storage device
characters per second	Speed measurement for computer printers
cursor	Flashing bar, arrow, or symbol that indicates where the next character will be placed
database	Computer application that contains files or records
data debugging	Process of eliminating errors from input data

(continued)

Table 2-1 (*Continued*)

Term	Definition
disk drive	A container that holds a read/write head, an access arm, and a magnetic disk for storage
downtime	The time a computer cannot be used due to maintenance or mechanical failure
e-mail	Use of a modem or direct-access dedicated line to transmit data electronically from computer to computer
file	A collection of related records
file maintenance	Data entry operations, including additions, modifications, and deletions
format	Methods for setting margins, line spacing, tabs, and other layout features
GIGO	"Garbage in, garbage out"—meaning that incorrect input will provide the incorrect output
hard copy	A printed copy of data in a file
hardware	The actual physical equipment used by a computer to process data
input	Entering data into a computer system
interface	Technology allowing nonconnected computers to exchange programs and data; also called a "network"
keyboard	An input device that resembles a typewriter keyboard

Table 2-1 *(Continued)*

Term	Definition
menu	A list of options available to users
modem	A hardware device that converts digital signals to analog signals for transfer over communication lines or links; modems are becoming less popular as direct-access lines eliminate the need for them
output	Processed data translated into the final form or information to be used
peripheral	Device required for input, output, processing, and storage of data; peripherals include the mouse, disk drive, printer, keyboard, and joystick
scrolling	Feature that allows the computer operator to control the location of the cursor within a document
security code	A group of characters allowing an authorized computer operator to access certain programs or features; also known as a "password"
write protect	Feature of storage devices allowing data to be seen but not changed

Computer Components

Computers are made up of *hardware* and *software*. Hardware includes items, such as the *monitor*, *keyboard*, and *printer*. The four main types of computer hardware are as follows:

• Input devices—allow the entering of data into computers; these include

- Keyboards—allow alphanumeric and other characters to be entered
- Pointing devices:
  - A *mouse* allows the user to move a *cursor*, viewed on a monitor, around the screen to specific areas. Items can be "clicked on" with the mouse to access or open them.
  - *Touch pads* are flat areas common on laptops and notebooks. They allow similar actions to be performed as with a mouse, but the user simply slides a finger across the touch pad.
  - *Touch screens* are special computer monitors that respond to the touch of a finger, pen, or a *wand*. They are becoming more popular in hospitals and clinical settings.
- Modems—transfer information between computers, using various types of wired lines. They are actually both input and output devices. They can be internal, external, or wireless.
  - *Cable modems*—operate over cable television lines
  - *Digital subscriber line (DSL) modems*—use telephone lines, but at different frequencies; they allow Internet access and telephone use at the same time
  - *Fax modems*—send and receive files similarly to fax machines, but are not as easily used since they involve the use of computer input and scanners
- Scanners—allow printed matter to be "scanned" and converted into a readable computer format; their use is much quicker than inputting information via a keyboard. They may be handheld, single-sheet scanners, or *flatbed scanners*, which resemble photocopiers.

Various computer components are shown in Figure 2-2.

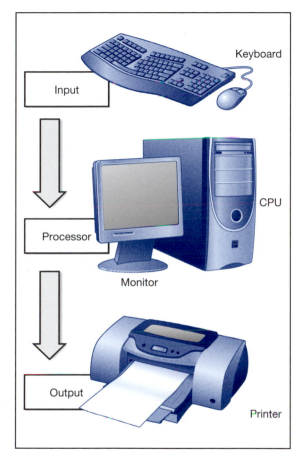

Keyboard

Input

CPU

Processor

Monitor

Output

Printer

Figure 2-2 *Components of a computer system.*

> **Key Focus:** Today's photocopiers have scanning capabilities and can transmit scanned documents directly into computers.

- Processing devices—include the *motherboard*, which controls the other components, and the *central processing unit (CPU)*, also known as the *microprocessor*. The CPU is the main computer chip that interprets all software program instructions.
- Storage devices—utilize computer *memory* to store information temporarily or permanently, and include
  - Random-access memory (RAM)—temporary, programmable memory; with more RAM available, the computer system performs faster
  - Read-only memory (ROM)—permanent memory that cannot be altered; the best example is the storage of computer operating systems in the form of ROM
  - Hard disk drives—store information permanently so that it can be retrieved when needed; larger hard disk drives allow for more storage of software programs and other information
  - Removable drives—used in addition to a computer's hard disk drive, and include
    - CD-ROM drives— "compact disc, read-only memory" drives that may be used either to import stored information or to save information to blank CD-R (recordable) discs
    - CD burners or recorders—allow copying of information from a CD or CD-R to another CD-R
    - External hard drives—often used as backup devices to an office's computers; they may also be used via Internet access to regularly back up files
    - Optical disc drives—utilize *digital video discs (DVDs)* to optically store information; their

advantage over CD-Rs is that they can store much greater amounts of data

- ○ USB flash drives—small devices, only about 2 inches in length, that can store many *gigabytes* of data; they attach to computers via *USB ports*
- ○ Zip drives—only rarely used today, primarily for backing up hard disks and transporting large files

- Output devices—used to display information after it has been processed; they include

  - Monitors—computer "screens" that display many types of information; today, monitors are thinner and flatter than in previous years, with better image resolution, helping to avoid eye strain
  - Printers—produce *hard copies* of files on paper, and include
    - ○ Laser printers—high-resolution, extremely fast printers that offer the highest quality; they use dry *toner* to print characters with extreme crispness and detail
    - ○ Inkjet printers—use small ink drops to print characters, and are more popular in smaller offices
  - Speakers—allow the user to hear computer-generated and other sounds

Computer *software* consists of sets of instructions that tell computers what functions to perform. The two basic categories are as follows:

- Operating system software—one example is *Windows*, used by Microsoft; operating system software is required by every computer in order to operate; *icons* are used, which are symbols representing specific functions such as printing, saving files, and performing various editing functions

- Application software—includes a large variety of different functions, as follows:
  - Word processing—allows writing of correspondence, reports, physician notes, and so on
  - Presentations—programs such as PowerPoint that create full-color informational "slides" that include text, graphics, audio, and video
  - Desktop publishing—creates documents with page layout formats, usually for printing of books and other printed materials
  - Spreadsheets—mostly used for accounting and billing, including financial reports and tax records; electronic transactions are handled easily, including credit card payments
  - Practice management—utilizes information *databases* to store patient records, medical charts, and insurance company information; it deals with day-to-day operations and scheduling
  - Optical character recognition (OCR)—allows images to be converted to text
  - Communications—allow for the use of e-mail, online discussion groups, up-to-date healthcare research information via medical database libraries, and other Internet activities

Advances in Computer Technology

Computer technology is advancing at a rapid rate. The following are some examples:

- Speech recognition—allows computers to interpret spoken words from the user through a microphone
- Telemedicine—use of telecommunications to transmit video images such as teleconferences with multiple healthcare providers, and CT scans and other types of imaging

Table 2-2 lists various medical resources found on the Internet.

Computer Security

Only authorized personnel should access confidential information. Computer *screensavers* should be used to prevent unauthorized viewing of information on monitors. It is important to *log off* or *lock* computers when they are not in use. Additional protective measures include

- Passwords—special codes, assigned to each computer user, that must be entered before access is allowed; never share passwords; if choosing your own, never use one that could easily be guessed by others; passwords are usually changed every 60 to 90 days, and include combinations of letters, numbers, and symbols
- Encryption software—encodes protected health information so that only users with passwords can open documents in their "decoded" format
- Activity-monitoring systems—used to record all users and their computer activities
- Antivirus software—protects computers from malicious software (viruses) that may attempt to corrupt files or steal data
- Firewalls—electronic barriers that keep unauthorized outsiders from gaining access to computer systems
- Computer disaster recovery plans—determine actions to be taken if a computer or system "crashes," meaning that all information becomes unavailable; they should include the following:
  - Automatic warnings—indicate fatal errors and provide directions to reduce information loss and damage to equipment
  - Regular backups—allow for information to be retrieved if a primary computer system crashes

Table 2-2 *Medical Resources on the Internet*

Source	Website	Comments
American Medical Association	https://www.ama-assn.org	Promotes the art and science of medicine and the betterment of public health.
eMedicineHealth	http://www.emedicinehealth.com	A consumer health information site with over 900 health and medical articles, with a focus on emergency medicine, written by physicians.
Health.gov	https://health.gov	The Office of Disease Prevention and Health Promotion (ODPHP) leads efforts to improve the health of all Americans.
MedlinePlus	https://medlineplus.gov	The National Institutes of Health's website for patients and their families and friends; produced by the National Library of Medicine.

National Institutes of Health	https://www.nih.gov	The nation's medical research agency—making important discoveries that improve health and save lives.
National Library of Medicine	https://www.nlm.nih.gov	A center of information innovation, and the world's largest biomedical library. It supports and conducts research, development, and training.
New England Journal of Medicine	http://www.nejm.org	Dedicated to bringing physicians the best research and key information about biomedical science and clinical practice.
WebMD Health	http://www.webmd.com	Provides valuable health information, tools for managing health, and support to people seeking information. Content is timely and credible.

- Safeguarding protected health information—steps to take to ensure protection of the privacy of patient records, using specified procedures that all staff members have been instructed on

Electronic Signatures

Electronic signatures use *encrypted characters*, which authenticate the identities of individuals who send documents or make agreements with other people. They hold legal significance, and are an important part of electronic health records. Electronic signatures are largely replacing traditional signatures on paper, written by hand.

Additional Equipment

Additional administrative equipment that may be used along with computers, and may even have certain computerized interactions or functions, includes

- Facsimile (fax) machines—scan documents and transmit them over telephone lines; they must be safeguarded because they may include PHI; fax cover sheets should be used containing a *disclaimer* that the fax is only for the intended receiver, and if received in error, must be destroyed, with the sender notified
- Photocopiers—reproduce all types of documents, using either dry toner or liquid ink
- Calculators and/or adding machines—calculators are usually portable and often battery or solar powered; adding machines usually are plugged into electrical outlets and produce paper tape on which calculations are printed
- Typewriters—rarely used today, usually to complete paper medical forms or envelopes
- Postal scales—used to weigh outgoing mail and determine amount of postage required

- Postage meters—used to apply printed postage amounts to envelopes or packages instead of stamps
- Folding and inserting machines—fold letters and insert materials into envelopes
- Dictations and transcription equipment—used to transcribe recorded words into written text
- Paper shredders—cut discarded documents into tiny pieces so that they cannot be read
- Check writers—machines that imprint checks instead of writing them manually; they interface with many different software packages

Maintenance of Office Equipment

Computers and other office equipment require regular maintenance, often on a weekly basis, but sometimes daily. Equipment manuals should be consulted for proper maintenance procedures. More complicated maintenance should be performed by the equipment suppliers, under the terms of their maintenance contracts. Before calling them

- First troubleshoot the problem to determine whether you can correct it yourself following the instruction manual.
- Consider using backup systems for specific pieces of equipment. Examples of backup devices include cell phones instead of traditional phones, emergency electrical generators, battery power backups, regular replacement of batteries in devices, and properly maintained fire extinguishers.

CHAPTER 3
Appointment Scheduling

A variety of factors may affect appointment scheduling, including

- Physician's preference
- Type and size of the physician's practice
- Availability of equipment
- Availability of staff
- Amount of flexibility required by the physician(s)
- Insurance coverage issues
- Patient needs
- Physician's schedule

APPOINTMENT TYPES

Two types of appointment scheduling systems include

1. Scheduled appointments
2. Open office hours

Key Focus: Some medical offices may offer extended evening hours or may be open 24 hours per day.

Types of scheduling:

- **Double booking**—scheduling two patients to be seen during the same time slot without allowing for any additional time in the schedule

Appointment Scheduling (vertical side tab)

- **Regular wave**—each hour is divided into four 15-minute segments, depending on how many patients can be seen within an hour, but all patients are told to come in at the beginning of the hour in which they are to be seen; they are seen in the order in which they arrive
- **Modified wave**—a flexible system built on the hour as the base of each block of time, allowing for the actual time used by patient appointments to average out over 1 hour
- **Open hour system**—patients may arrive at any time during open hours
- **Procedure grouping**—many physicians prefer to have similar procedures and examinations scheduled during a particular block of time
- **Cluster scheduling**—similar appointments together on a specific day, or for a specific block of time during the day or week
- **Advance scheduling**—patients might be booked weeks or months in advance

APPOINTMENT CONFIRMATIONS

Several types of appointment reminders are used to help patients keep track of their appointments:
- Confirmation calls
- E-mail notifications
- Reminder mailings
- Appointment cards

PATIENT SCHEDULING SITUATIONS

Medical assistants must deal with special situations that arise regarding the scheduling of patients. Examples include
- Emergencies
- Fasting patients

- Referrals
- Late arrivals
- Walk-ins
- Diabetic patients
- Cancellations

SCHEDULING SYSTEMS

Appointment scheduling facilitates the coordination of appropriate time segments for staff, patients, and the practice's available equipment. Appointment systems may be kept electronically or manually.

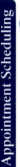

> **Key Focus:** Appointment documentation is considered a legal document in litigation.

Computerized Systems

Computerized appointment systems are very commonly used today; Health Insurance Portability and Accountability Act of 1996 (HIPAA) guidelines must be followed.

Computer security techniques include

- Accessibility requirements (including controls to allow only appropriate personnel to view certain patient information)
- Proper firewalls
- Confidentiality
- Employee computer authorization
- Positioning and locating monitors for staff visibility only
- Changing of employee passwords frequently

Advantages of computerized scheduling include

- The ability to "lock out" specific areas for designated reasons, such as emergency or last-minute appointments

- Access of information from multiple areas inside the office
- Identification of "problem patients" due to no-shows, late arrivals, or cancellations
- Searching for upcoming appointments in order to provide adequate follow-up care
- Creating reports on the office's overall scheduling activities
- Color-coding, used to help visually identify areas designated for specific types of appointments
- Searching for requested available times or days

Online Scheduling

Online scheduling is also known as *e-scheduling*, and is becoming more popular. It allows patients to schedule their own appointments or request appointments by using the Internet. Over time, costs have decreased and security measures have improved for online scheduling. Although setup time and staff training are required, online scheduling can greatly improve the scheduling process. It is important to determine whether it will benefit the practice first.

COMMON ABBREVIATIONS FOR SCHEDULING

BP—blood pressure check
can/cx—cancellation
CDE or CPE—complete diagnostic exam/complete physical exam
c/o—complains of
cons—consultation
CP—chest pain
ECG/EKG—electrocardiogram
FBS—fasting blood sugar
F/u, f/u, or F/U—follow-up
I&D—incision and drainage

inj—injection
lab—laboratory studies
minor surg—minor surgery
N&V—nausea and vomiting
NP—new patient
NS—no-show patient
P&P—pelvic (exam) and Pap (smear)
Pap—Pap smear
pt—patient
PT—physical therapy
RBS—random blood sugar
re—recheck
ref—referral
RS—reschedule
Rx—prescription
Sig—sigmoidoscopy
S/R—suture removal
surg—surgery
US or U/S—ultrasound

SCHEDULING PROCESS

Steps that should be taken include the following:

- Gather and organize all required equipment
- Utilize effective communication skills

Table 3-1 lists time estimates for specific office procedures.

Key Focus: If the medical practice has a cancellation charge for a no-show, the patient must be made aware of the policy prior to cancellation. It is often preferable for a patient to cancel his or her appointment ahead of time rather than just not show up.

Table 3-1 *Time Estimates for Specific Office Procedures*

Procedure	Minutes of Time
Allergy testing	30–60
Blood pressure check	15
Cast check	10
Cast change	30
Complete physical with EKG	60
Dressing change	15
Minor surgery procedure	30–45
Office visit: Established patient	
Low complexity	5–10
Medium complexity	15–20
High complexity	20–30
Office visit: New patient	
Low complexity	10–15
Medium complexity	15–30
Complete physical	30–45
Patient education	30–45
Pelvic examination with Pap test	30
Postoperative checkup	15–20
Prenatal checkup	15
Prenatal examination (first visit)	30–60
Prostate examination	30
School physical	15–30
Suture removal	10
Well-baby checkup	15

Note: EKG, electrocardiogram; Pap, Papanicolaou.

EMERGENCY APPOINTMENTS

In order to eliminate the need to "squeeze in" emergency or nonscheduled appointments (and possibly disrupt the time management office flow), the medical assistant should set time patterns. Time patterns are periods within the schedule for catch-up time or nonscheduled appointments. It is important to build small blocks of time into the schedule during the day when the physician can do the following:

- Return telephone calls
- Catch up on charting
- Read mail and journals
- Rest

"Buffer" periods are excellent times for emergencies that may have to be seen that day. Examples of emergency conditions in the medical office are

- Acute allergic reactions
- Convulsions
- Diabetic reactions
- Fever over 104°F
- Foreign objects in the eyes
- Fractures
- Head injuries
- Lacerations
- Near-drowning (ingestion of water into the lungs)
- Pain or numbness after application of a cast for a fracture
- Severe dizziness
- Severe pain
- Sudden acute illness

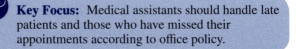

Key Focus: Medical assistants should handle late patients and those who have missed their appointments according to office policy.

NEW PATIENT APPOINTMENTS

The following steps are guidelines for scheduling a new patient:

- Obtain the patient's full legal name with correct spelling, birth date, full address, telephone number, and e-mail address
- Record the patient's chief complaints and symptoms
- Request the name of the patient's insurance carrier and policy number
- Ask the patient for a preferred appointment time and attempt to accommodate it
- Confirm the day, date, and time of the appointment
- Provide directions to the office
- Inform new patients that they should bring the following:
  - Insurance verification
  - Photo identification
  - A list of current medications, current laboratory reports, x-rays, and other medical reports (as available)
- Document new patient information in the computer or in a new written medical record

APPOINTMENTS OUTSIDE THE MEDICAL OFFICE

Medical assistants are often required to make appointments for patients outside the medical office. These may include appointments for

- Laboratory work
- Radiology
- ECG and stress testing
- Inpatient and outpatient surgeries
- Hospital admission
- Referrals to other physicians

CHAPTER 4
Mail Processing and Managing Correspondence

Medical assistants are responsible for mail processing and managing correspondence.

Common items in the daily mail include the following:

- Advertisements
- Bills
- Correspondence
- Hospital and physician reports
- Insurance forms
- Laboratory results and reports
- Mailings from medical societies and other medical professional organizations
- Patient payments
- Medical journals
- Promotional drug information and samples

Key Focus: The physician may choose to personally open any financial or legal piece of mail, even when they are not marked "personal."

INCOMING MAIL

Medical assistants must handle incoming mail, which is very important for the office, patients, and other professionals. The processes of handling incoming mail involve the following steps:

- Sorting
- Opening

- Recording
- Annotating
- Distributing

> **Key Focus:** Many physicians receive a number of drug samples in the mail. The medical assistant must ensure that all drug samples received are stored in a locked cabinet.

PROCEDURE 4-1 *Opening the Mail*

Medical assistants must sort the mail that arrives in the medical office daily using the following equipment and supplies:

- Computer
- Date stamp
- Paper, pens, and pencils
- Highlighters
- Office letterhead and envelopes
- Letter opener
- Paper clips
- Stapler
- Staple remover

Method

1. Clear a working space on the desk.
2. Sort the mail by its importance into the following categories: the physician's personal mail, first-class mail, insurance company mail, patient payments, magazines and newspapers, drug samples, and miscellaneous mail.
3. Stack all envelopes so that they are facing in the same direction and tap each envelope so that the contents

settle toward the bottom to avoid cutting the contents with the letter opener.

4. Open all envelopes along the top edge.
5. Be sure everything is removed from each envelope.
6. When needed, take note of the postmark.
7. Before discarding any envelopes, be sure the contents include a return address.
8. Stamp each letter with the date and attach any enclosures that came with the letter.
9. If an enclosure was indicated as being included in the envelope with a letter, but it was not in the envelope, you should write the word "no" beside the listed enclosure and circle the enclosure that is missing.

Key Focus: Each office has its own specific requirements for the way that mail is sorted. Medical assistants should always follow their office's policies and procedures first.

BUSINESS LETTERS

A business letter includes

- Heading: letterhead, such as the physician's or the practice's name, address, telephone number
- Date: month, day, year
- Inside address: who receives the correspondence
- Salutation: a courteous greeting
- Body: containing the purpose of the letter
- Closing: containing a courteous ending word
- Reference initials: who typed the letter
- Enclosure notation: indicating whether other documents are included with the letter
- Cc (carbon copy): indicates people who are receiving copies of the letter

Letter Styles

- Block
- Modified block (standard)
- Modified block with indented paragraphs
- Simplified
- Semi-simplified

Please see Figure 4-1 for some examples of letter styles.

MAIL NEEDING SPECIAL HANDLING

- Drug samples—new samples must be kept in a storage area, arranged by expiration date. Drugs should always be sorted before they are placed in containers.
- Insurance information—to avoid a delay in payment, documents should be given to the appropriate person right away.
- Payment receipts—all payments should be sorted and then recorded.
- Vacation mail—when the physician is out of the office, the medical assistant must decide how to handle the mail and must evaluate any mail that might need the physician's immediate attention.

Key Focus: Confidentiality is of the utmost importance, and medical assistants must keep this in mind regarding the opening of mail in the physician's office.

OUTGOING MAIL

Steps when sending mail:

- Fold and insert letters into envelopes
- Address envelopes completely

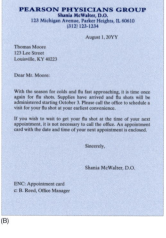

Figure 4-1 *Letter styles: (A) block, (B) modified block.*

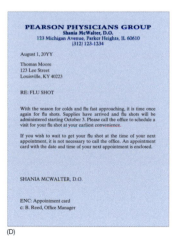

PEARSON PHYSICIANS GROUP
Shania McWalter, D.O.
123 Michigan Avenue, Parker Heights, IL 60610
(312) 123-1234

August 1, 20YY

Thomas Moore
123 Lee Street
Louisville, KY 40223

Dear Mr. Moore:

    With the season for colds and flu fast approaching, it is time once again for flu shots. Supplies have arrived and flu shots will be administered starting October 3. Please call the office to schedule a visit for your flu shot at your earliest convenience.

    If you wish to wait to get your flu shot at the time of your next appointment, it is not necessary to call the office. An appointment card with the date and time of your next appointment is enclosed.

               Sincerely,

               Shania McWalter, D.O.

ENC: Appointment card
c: B. Reed, Office Manager

(C)

PEARSON PHYSICIANS GROUP
Shania McWalter, D.O.
123 Michigan Avenue, Parker Heights, IL 60610
(312) 123-1234

August 1, 20YY

Thomas Moore
123 Lee Street
Louisville, KY 40223

RE: FLU SHOT

With the season for colds and flu fast approaching, it is time once again for flu shots. Supplies have arrived and flu shots will be administered starting October 3. Please call the office to schedule a visit for your flu shot at your earliest convenience.

If you wish to wait to get your flu shot at the time of your next appointment, it is not necessary to call the office. An appointment card with the date and time of your next appointment is enclosed.

SHANIA MCWALTER, D.O.

ENC: Appointment card
c: B. Reed, Office Manager

(D)

Figure 4-1 *Letter styles: (C) modified block with indented paragraphs, and (D) simplified.*

Alabama	AL	Montana	MT
Alaska	AK	Nebraska	NE
Arizona	AZ	Nevada	NV
Arkansas	AR	New Hampshire	NH
California	CA	New Jersey	NJ
Canal Zone	CZ	New Mexico	NM
Colorado	CO	New York	NY
Connecticut	CT	North Carolina	NC
Delaware	DE	North Dakota	ND
District of Columbia	DC	Ohio	OH
Florida	FL	Oklahoma	OK
Georgia	GA	Oregon	OR
Guam	GU	Pennsylvania	PA
Hawaii	HI	Puerto Rico	PR
Idaho	ID	Rhode Island	RI
Illinois	IL	South Carolina	SC
Indiana	IN	South Dakota	SD
Iowa	IA	Tennessee	TN
Kansas	KS	Texas	TX
Kentucky	KY	Utah	UT
Louisiana	LA	Vermont	VT
Maine	ME	Virgin Islands	VI
Maryland	MD	Virginia	VA
Massachusetts	MA	Washington	WA
Michigan	MI	West Virginia	WV
Minnesota	MN	Wisconsin	WI
Mississippi	MS	Wyoming	WY
Missouri	MO		

Figure 4-2 *Two-letter abbreviations for the United States and territories.*

- Write the return address on each envelope
- Make any needed notes on each envelope such as "personal" or "confidential"
- Seal and stamp each envelope
- Use the two-digit letter abbreviation for states (see Figure 4-2)
- Stamp the correct postage

Classifications of Mail

Mail is classified depending upon type, weight, and destination. Table 4-1 explains these classifications.

Table 4-1 *Mail Classifications*

Type	Description
First class	Letters, postcards, business reply cards; letters weighing less than 11 ounces; sealed and unsealed, handwritten or typed material
Priority	First-class mail weighing more than 11 ounces; maximum weight of 70 pounds; postage calculated based on weight and destination
Second class	Newspapers and periodicals that have received second-class mail authorization; copies of newspapers and periodicals mailed by the general public who are not able to receive the second-class rate
Third class	Catalogs, books, photographs, flyers, and other printed materials (also called "bulk mail"); must be marked "Third Class"; must be sealed *(continued)*

Table 4-1 (*Continued*)

Type	Description
Fourth class	Printed material, books, and merchandise not included in first and second class; must weigh between 16 ounces and 70 pounds; there are size limitations also
Express mail/next day service	Available 7 days a week; up to 70 pounds in weight and 108 inches around; expected delivery by noon; shipping containers are supplied; pickup service in some areas

Special Postal Services

Table 4-2 describes special postal services.

Table 4-2 *Special Postal Services*

Type	Description
Certified mail	Mail that is not valuable itself, but difficult to replace if lost (birth certificates, contracts, etc.)
Special delivery	When fast delivery of an item is needed; it is useful for shipping perishable items
Special handling	Can be requested for third- and fourth-class items

Table 4-2 (*Continued*)

Type	Description
Forwarding mail	If the incorrect address is crossed out, the new address is inserted, and the mail is returned to the mail carrier or Post Office, it will be forwarded to the new address for up to 6 months
Mail recall	If mail was placed into a mailbox or given to a carrier by mistake, it can be recalled by the sender
Tracing mail	If mail did not arrive after a normal period of time, the Post Office will try to trace it for the sender
Returned mail	Mail returned or marked "undeliverable" cannot be re-marked or re-sent until new postage is added
Insured mail	Insurance can be purchased for third-class, fourth-class, or priority mail. The sender will then be reimbursed for the content if this mail is lost or damaged
Postal money orders	Can be bought and sent in place of cash or checks; can also be replaced if lost or stolen
Collect on delivery (COD)	Used if the sender wants to collect payment for postage from the recipient when the mail is delivered

(*continued*)

Mail Processing

Table 4-2 *(Continued)*

Type	Description
Private delivery services	Many private services offer various delivery options, even delivering mail overnight
Restricted delivery	Delivered only to a specific addressee or to someone authorized in writing to receive mail for the addressee; this is available only for registered, certified, or COD mail, or mail insured for more than $50
Delivery confirmation	Mail is tracked using a tracking number, by its delivery date, and by signature of the recipient

CHAPTER 5
Medical Records Management

Medical records provide a continuous story of a patient's progress from the first visit to the last, with all essential information, observations, illnesses, treatments, and outcomes carefully documented.

THE IMPORTANCE OF MEDICAL RECORDS

Medical records provide

- Continuity in a patient's medical care—this helps develop a "Patient Care Partnership"
- Statistical information
- Better quality of treatment
- Documentation for malpractice cases and lawsuits
- Documentation for insurance billing and defending audits by managed care companies, Medicare, Medicaid

Standard Medical Records

Medical records generally include the following information:

- Address and phone number of the patient
- Informed consent forms
- Medical history of the patient
- Family history (Fx)
- Occupational history
- Insurance
- Chief complaint (CC)
- Physical examination results
- Progress notes

- Laboratory reports
- Operative reports
- X-ray reports
- EKG
- Medications
- Discharge summaries

TYPES OF MEDICAL RECORDS

The most common formats of medical records are as follows:

- **Source-oriented medical record (SOMR)**, also called the *conventional method*:
  - Uses areas of data from the patient, treating physician, specialist, laboratory, hospital, and so on
- **Problem-oriented medical record (POMR)**—easier to track patient's progress:
  - Database—includes a record of the patient's past medical history
  - Problem list—each condition or diagnosis is listed separately and uniquely numbered
  - Educational, diagnostic, and treatment plan—diagnoses, treatments, and patient instructions
  - Progress notes—chronologically list conditions, complaints, problems, treatments, and responses

Many offices using the POMR format emphasize **SOAP documentation**:

- **S**—*subjective* data from the patient, describing signs and symptoms, with opinions and comments
- **O**—*objective* data from the physician, examinations, and test results
- **A**—*assessment:* the diagnosis or impression of the patient's problem

- **P**—*plan of action:* treatment options, selected treatment, medications, tests, consultations, patient education, and follow-up

> **Key Focus:** SOAP documentation can be used regardless of whether the office utilizes SOMR or POMR charting.

A further way to break down SOAP documentation is with the **CHEDDAR format**:

- **C**—*chief complaint:* presents problems and subjective statements
- **H**—*history:* medical, family, and social histories, history of presenting problem (HPI), and so on
- **E**—*examination:* details about the body systems that were examined
- **D**—*details:* of problem and complaints
- **D**—*drugs and dosage:* list of current medications, with dosages and frequency of administration
- **A**—*assessment:* of diagnostic process, with impression (diagnosis) by the practitioner
- **R**—*return* visit information, or referral, if required

ELECTRONIC MEDICAL RECORDS

Electronic medical records (EMR) software allows you to create, store, edit, and retrieve patient charts on a computer. Paper charts can then be replaced with electronic charts. The computer-based medical record (or *electronic health record*) is much more efficient than paper-based records, and is becoming more common. Most outpatient medical practices use computers for

keeping patient information and conducting various
activities, including

- Demographic data
- Insurance billing
- Printing statements
- Posting payments
- Scheduling and appointments
- Word processing
- Accounting and tracking
- Computer charting

All data are saved, backed up, and stored electronically.

Security of EMR

The Health Insurance Portability and Accountability
Act of 1996 (HIPAA) was passed to ensure the privacy
of patients' records when transferring information
between health professionals, which might decrease the
quality of care. To provide security, you must do the
following:

- Keep all computer backup disks in a safe place.
- Store disks in a bank safe-deposit box.
- Use passwords with characters other than letters and
  encrypt the passwords.
- Change login codes and passwords every 30 days.
- Turn terminals away from areas where information may
  be seen by patients.
- Keep fax machines and printers that receive personal
  medical information in a private place.
- Ensure that each user is restricted to the information
  needed to do his or her job.
- Train staff members about confidentiality and each
  person's responsibility.

- Appoint a specific security officer to oversee the security of EMR.
- Provide a written confidentiality policy that employees must sign.
- Conduct routine audits and disciplinary measures for breaches of confidentiality.

RECORDS MANAGEMENT

The objectives of good medical records management include

- Reducing misfiles
- Complying with legal safeguards
- Retrieving information more quickly
- Saving time for the physician, staff, and patient
- Reducing filing equipment expenditures
- Saving space

Key Focus: Patients own the information in their medical records, but the facility that created this information owns the physical or electronic medical records.

The Six Cs of Charting

There are six Cs of charting, in order to maintain accurate patient records:

- Clients (patients)
- Clarity
- Completeness
- Conciseness
- Chronological order
- Confidentiality

Auditing Medical Records

The process of auditing involves periodic examining and reviewing groups of patient records, making sure that they are complete and accurate. This is very important so that they "back up" charges that were sent to health insurance companies for reimbursement. There are two types of audits:

- Internal audits—performed by the medical staff or by hired *compliance specialists*. Patient records are randomly chosen, with audits performed at two times:
  - Before billing is submitted (*prospective*)
  - After billing is submitted (*retrospective*)
- External audits—performed by government entities such as Medicare or Medicaid, private insurance carriers, and managed care organizations (MCOs). These audits have become more common due to federal and private organizations attempting to recover overpayments. External audits may result in

  - Interviews of staff members, patients, and healthcare providers
  - Charges of fraud when medical records do not back up charges submitted for payment
  - Returns of payments to payers or patients if found to be fraudulent
  - Possible severe financial penalties, loss of participation in federal programs, imprisonment, and loss of license to practice

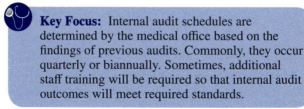

Key Focus: Internal audit schedules are determined by the medical office based on the findings of previous audits. Commonly, they occur quarterly or biannually. Sometimes, additional staff training will be required so that internal audit outcomes will meet required standards.

Files or Records

There are three categories of files or records in the medical office:

- Active records—patients currently seeing the physician
- Inactive records—patients who have not seen the physician for 3 years (each office will have its own policy for moving a record to "inactive")
- Closed records—patients who are no longer seeing the physician or have died

Filing Equipment

- Compactable files—for small offices
- Automated files—require more upkeep than others
- Rotary circular files—hold many records
- Shelf files—should have doors
- Lateral files—common in physician's own offices
- Drawer files—may have a locking device

Key Focus: All records should be stored in a fireproof, waterproof area that is locked when not in use.

Filing Procedures

There are six steps involved in filing:

- Conditioning (or inspecting)—removing paper clips or fasteners, stapling related papers together, attaching smaller papers to full-size sheets with rubber cement or tape, and fixing damaged records
- Releasing—placing a mark on sheets' upper-left corners to indicate readiness for filing (usually the word FILE or the medical assistant's initials)

- Indexing—separating items to be filed by assigning certain information to numbered fields or units (patient's last name, then first name, then middle initial, then title or special designation)
- Coding—placing an indication of how the file will be indexed on the sheets; often, the name or subject is underlined; all sheets should have the date and patient's name on them, usually in upper right-hand corner
- Sorting—arranging sheets to be filed sequentially, by removing loose pieces or tape or paper clips
- Storing and filing—placing items face up with the top edge to the left, and the most recent date at the front of the folder; the folders should be listed a few inches out of the drawer before new material is inserted; it is preferred that new items are permanently attached to the correct file folder; completed folders should be arranged in indexing order before re-filing

FILING SYSTEMS

Basic methods of filing include

- Alphabetic filing—the most common system (rules for alphabetic filing are listed in Appendix D)

Key Focus: The key to alphabetical filing is to divide the names and titles into units (first, second, and third). The unit is the portion of the name that is used for filing or indexing purposes.

- Subject filing—may be used for general files, such as the following:
  - Invoices
  - Correspondence

- Resumes
- Personnel records
- Numeric filing—used in hospitals and larger clinics and requires the use of an alphabetical cross-reference to locate a file. This is generally a six-digit number divided into three sections of two digits each (such as 03-85-42). Several types of numeric filing include the following:
  - Unit numbering
  - Straight numeric filing: patients are assigned consecutive numbers as they visit
  - Filing by terminal digit: patients are also given consecutive numbers, but the digits in the number are usually separated into groups and are read from right to left; these records are filed backward
  - Middle digit filing: begins with the middle digits, then the first digit, and then the last digit
  - Serial numbering
- Phonetic filing—used primarily for the classification of names. Phonetic systems assign numerical values to different letter sounds. This allows file searches for names that may sound similar but may be spelled differently.

Labeling

- Each file must be labeled to identify the name of the patient.
- Labels are also used to identify each shelf, drawer, and divider guide.

Color-Coding Filing

Helps to locate a specific chart more easily by using color in numeric or alphabetic filing systems.

Numerical Color Coding

Separate colors are assigned for each number (from zero to nine), with color bars on the end of each file corresponding to the medical record number. Usually, only three primary digits are color-coded. The Ames Color File System and the Smead Manufacturing Company System are commonly used numerical filing systems (see Table 5-1).

Alphabetical Color Coding

The Smead Manufacturing Company also makes a popular alphabetical color-coded system known as "Alpha-Z" that is based on 13 different colors that are

Table 5-1 *Numerical Color-Coding Systems*

Ames Color File System	Smead Manufacturing Company
0–red	0–yellow
1–gray	1–blue
2–blue	2–pink
3–orange	3–purple
4–purple	4–orange
5–black	5–brown
6–yellow	6–green
7–brown	7–gray
8–pink	8–red
9–green	9–black

Table 5-2 *Alpha-Z Alphabetic Color-Coding System*

Color	White Letter, No Stripe	White Letter, White Stripe
Red	A	N
Dark blue	B	O
Dark green	C	P
Light blue	D	Q
Purple	E	R
Orange	F	S
Gray	G	T
Dark brown	H	U
Pink	I	V
Yellow	J	W
Light brown	K	X
Lavender	L	Y
Light green	M	Z

Medical Records

used for the first 13 letters of the alphabet. For the second 13 letters of the alphabet, this system uses the same 13 colors but with a white stripe added to differentiate them (see Table 5-2).

Tickler Files
A tickler file is a date-ordered reminder file that helps avoid losing track of important dates. Examples include entering of reminders to order supplies, or to send patient checkups.

Locating Missing Files

The best method to avoid losing a file is to file all records carefully and methodically. Guidelines to help you locate missing files include

- Looking for look-alike or sound-alike names, such as Klein and Kline.
- Looking for alternate spellings, such as Thompson or Tompson.
- Finding color-coded files that are misfiled with those that have the same color coding.
- Finding numeric file numbers that are misfiled due to transposition of numbers, such as 349201 and 394201.
- Finding alphabetic file names that are misfiled due to transposition of letters, such as Deitz and Dietz.
- Checking for other patient files that may have been filed on the same day.
- Finding missing files on the desks of the physician, billing clerk, and other office staff who may have had interaction with the missing file, as well as the "in" and "out" baskets used throughout the office.
- Putting in a placeholder for charts that have been removed from the filing cabinet.

CHAPTER 6
Forms of Communication

A medical assistant should be an effective communicator. This requires both clear verbal (spoken and written) and nonverbal (tone and body language) communication. Communication may include

- Creating a warm, reassuring environment
- Using proper telephone techniques
- Responding to or writing telephone messages
- Explaining procedures to patients
- Answering patients' questions
- Assisting physicians in a variety of procedures
- Assisting in billing issues
- Expediting insurance referral requests

TYPES OF COMMUNICATION

Communication may be positive or negative, verbal or nonverbal.

Positive Communication

- Be friendly and personable
- Give patients your full attention; listen carefully
- Never interrupt
- Speak slowly and clearly
- Ask questions if you do not understand
- Face the person as you speak
- Show empathy (identify with patient's feelings)
- Smile as you talk or listen
- Avoid terms that increase patient's anxiety

Key Focus: Patients vary in the amount of eye contact that makes them comfortable or uncomfortable.

Negative Communication

- No eye contact when speaking
- Interrupting before a person has finished speaking
- Mumbling when you are speaking
- Not using common conversational courtesies
- Explaining too rapidly confuses the listener
- Showing boredom when another person is speaking
- Speaking abruptly or harshly
- Treating patients in an impersonal manner makes you seem uncaring toward them

Key Focus: Religion and spirituality are common sources of miscommunication. Some people refuse to have blood drawn because they believe the process may bring bad luck or even cause death. Medical assistants must understand patients' diversities and adapt communicative procedures as needed.

Verbal Communication

Verbal communication consists of words, sounds, and voice tone, which are all important in conveying a message. You must select the right words, with the positive attitude, whenever you speak.

Nonverbal Communication

- Maintaining personal space
- Listening (this is extremely important)
- Eye contact (also very important)
- Appearance (physical features, clothing, grooming)
- Facial expressions
- Open posture is considered positive; closed posture is considered negative
- Touching (influenced by family background, age, gender, culture)

> **Key Focus:** Touching is not always acceptable depending on a person's culture and personal preference.

Defense Behaviors

A defensive behavior is a reaction to a perceived threat that is usually unconscious. This reaction may display the defense mechanisms outlined in Table 6-1.

> **Key Focus:** Body language can convey a person's true feelings, even when his or her words may indicate different or opposite feelings.

Ineffective Communication

Types of communication that may interfere with your communication style are outlined in Table 6-2.

Table 6-1 *Defense Mechanisms*

Mechanism	Definition
Compensation	Covering up weaknesses by emphasizing a more desirable trait
Denial	Ignoring unacceptable realities by refusing to acknowledge them
Displacement	Transferring of emotional reactions from one object to another
Dissociation	Removing emotional significance from ideas or events
Identification	Managing anxiety by imitating behavior of someone feared or respected
Introjection	Identification of others' values, even when contrary to one's previous assumptions
Projection	Blame is placed on others for unacceptable desires, thoughts, shortcomings, and mistakes
Rationalization	Justification of behaviors by faulty logic
Regression	Resorting to an earlier, more comfortable level of functioning
Repression	Threatening feelings and thoughts are kept hidden from consciousness
Substitution	Replacement of something unacceptable with something acceptable

Table 6-2 *Ineffective Communication*

Communication	Negative Implications
Reassuring	May make the patient feel that there is no need to worry
Approval	May lead to the patient striving for praise
Disapproving	May imply that you are judging the patient
Agreeing/disagreeing	May encourage or discourage the patient incorrectly
Advising	May put you outside your scope of practice
Probing	May involve discussing a topic the patient does not want to discuss
Defending	May cause the patient to end communication
Requesting explanations	May intimidate patients; avoid asking "why" because it may make a patient defensive
Minimizing	May cause the patients to feel that you are making light of them
Stereotyping	Uses meaningless statements in place of reasonable explanations

Forms of Communication

COMMUNICATING WITH DIFFERENT PATIENTS

Recognize each patient's needs and show empathy in allowing how he or she feels to ensure good communication. Ask the patient if you can help before doing so.

Communicating with Children

- Use dolls, pictures, and other models.
- Let them speak at own pace, completing sentences.
- Encourage children to talk about themselves.
- Use words that they easily understand.
- Recognize upsetting situations; be reassuring.
- Allow them to handle safe medical equipment such as stethoscopes.
- Sit at eye level, even on the floor if needed.

Communicating with the Geriatric Population

- Additional time may be required to communicate with older adults; display patience.
- Empathy acknowledges their age-related changes.
- Allow patients with hearing aids to adjust volume.
- Speak in a normal level, close enough to be heard.
- Never raise your voice.
- Be careful of body language.
- Speak clearly and slowly; avoid long explanations.
- Wait patiently for their responses.

Communicating with Patients

Patients may have difficulty seeing or hearing, or be otherwise physically or mentally disabled.

Communicating with Visually Disabled Patients

- Make patients comfortable in the unfamiliar surroundings of the office.
- Always explain what you will do and alert them before touching.
- Prevent patients from falling by providing verbal directions to avoid objects.
- Keep voice volume normal so that they are reassured and not threatened.

Communicating with Patients Who Have Difficulty Hearing

- Face patients directly when speaking.
- Touch the patients' arm or shoulder to alert them to face you before speaking.
- Speak clearly in a natural tone at a normal rate of speech; avoid shouting.
- Use hand gestures and facial expressions as communication cues.
- Use visual examples and reading materials.
- Involve friends or family by providing them with information for the patient.
- Minimize environmental distractions.

Key Focus: For the purpose of protecting yourself legally, you must consider the confidentiality of the patient's information, as well as patient needs such as hearing, language, or vision disabilities, and age-specific needs.

COMMUNICATING WITH COWORKERS

Some rules for communicating in the medical office include the following:

- Do not go to a supervisor before discussing the problem with the coworker first.
- A positive attitude will help you avoid conflict and resolve most problems.
- Schedule a good time to discuss an important topic; this ensures that the person you need to speak to can give the topic full attention.

Communicating with Superiors

- Superiors should be informed before problems can intensify.
- If you have a question for a superior, you should ask them.
- Show initiative and have well-outlined ideas.
- Make sure that your superior has enough time to talk.

SECTION II

Office Equipment and Financial Management

Office
Equipment

Chapter 7
Managing Supplies and Banking

The medical assistant is often responsible for ordering various equipment or supplies. Purchasing for the medical office requires research, evaluation, comparison, leasing, operation, and maintenance of essential equipment. Supplies refer to durable or expendable items. The medical assistant is also often responsible for banking procedures.

DURABLE ITEMS

Durable equipment consists of items that cost more money to purchase (generally over $500 in most offices) and have a relatively long life. These items are also referred to as "capital equipment." Examples include

- Autoclaves
- Computers (laptops and desktops)
- Fax machines
- Telephone system
- Copy machines and color laser printers
- Postage meters
- Refrigerators
- X-ray machines
- ECG machines
- Examination tables

Key Focus: Durable equipment has a financial life, which is referred to as *depreciation*. Depreciation is a loss in value of the product resulting from normal aging, use, and deterioration.

CONSUMABLE ITEMS

Examples of consumable, or expendable, items include

- Bandages
- Irrigating kits
- Prescription pads
- Rubber gloves

SUPPLIES

- *General office supplies*
  - Stationery: appointment cards and bookkeeping supplies
  - Pens, pencils, and erasers
  - Stamps
  - Staplers and staple removers
  - Insurance forms
  - Printer cartridges
  - CD-ROMs
  - Clipboards
  - File folders
  - Liquid soap
- *Clinical equipment*
  - Disposable speculums
  - Tongue blades
  - Disposable ear and nose covers for scopes
  - Disposable covers for thermometers
  - Cotton-tipped applicators
  - Elastic bandages
  - Lubricants
  - Needles
  - Syringes
  - Gloves
  - Goggles
  - Dressings

- Suture materials
- Sterilization bags and tapes
- *Paper supplies*
  - Examination table paper
  - Paper towels
  - Facial and toilet tissue
  - Paper cups
  - Disposable gowns
  - Drapes
  - Photocopy paper
  - Insurance and chart forms
  - Laboratory order forms
  - Appointment books
  - ECG paper
  - Receipt books
  - Appointment cards
- Current CPT and ICD-10 coding books

According to the urgency of need, supplies are also categorized into the following:

- Vital supplies, including prescription pads, needles, and syringes
- Incidental supplies, including stamps and staples
- Periodic supplies, including paper cups, disposable gowns, and ECG paper

Ordering Supplies

The ordering and checking of supplies, as well as dealing with vendors, help to avoid mistakes. In efficiently purchasing supplies for your office, the following steps must be followed:

- Collecting the prices of various vendors
- Making sure that the office spends between 4% and 6% of its annual gross income on administrative, clerical,

and general supplies; any more than this is excessive and detrimental to the cash flow of the office

- *Petty cash* is paper money and coins kept on hand to aid in transactions. Examples of petty cash include postage, cash payments, and minor purchases needed quickly. Most offices keep $50 to $100 of petty cash on hand.

Ordering Procedures

The medical assistant may be asked to research and compare equipment based on

- Manufacturer
- Quality
- Size
- Service
- Price
- Other determining factors

Standard practices for ordering and purchasing supplies:

- An authorized person should be in charge of purchasing
- High-quality goods and services should be ordered at the lowest prices available
- Paperwork should be fully and correctly completed
- Received orders should contain
  - *Packing slips*, usually without prices listed; explaining items and quantities included
    - Date received and quantity of each item are recorded on an inventory card or inventory record

This information must be checked against the order form that was created when the items were ordered. It must also be checked against the packing slip, dated with the actual received date, and initialed by the person doing the checking.

- Errors in shipments should be corrected

- Payments should be made in a timely manner
- Paid invoices should be kept on file
  - Invoices are requests for payment to a buyer, from a seller—including prices of items or services

Equipment Records
Medical assistants must maintain records of all office equipment:
- Receipts for major purchases
- Instruction and operating manuals
- Lists of service people with contact information

Payment
Payment may be made in the following ways:
- Cash
- Check
- Money order
- Credit card

BANKING FUNCTIONS

Medical assistants may be responsible for maintaining and controlling the medical office's banking and bookkeeping procedures. For handling banking, you may
- Accept checks
- Endorse checks
- Prepare and make deposits daily
- Compare total on deposit slip against day sheet
- Keep duplicate copy of all deposits filed in office
- Write checks
- Withdraw funds
- Maintain records of daily receipts in a safe location
- Immediately note all deposits in checkbook

Checks

A check is a payable, written order to a bank to pay or transfer money. *Types of checks include*

- Cashier's checks—guaranteed by a bank, using bank funds, and signed by a cashier
- Certified checks—sufficient funds for these checks are verified by a bank when they are written
- Money orders—payment orders for prespecified amounts of money
- Limited checks—restrict the amount to a specific maximum listed on them
- Traveler's checks—used in place of cash when traveling, and have preprinted amounts
- Voucher checks—have stubs for the payee, a record for the payer; used for specific purchases, in exact amounts
- Warrants—government checks payable on demand that are drawn by the government, or on the government

Key Focus: To prevent theft, checks should be endorsed "for deposit only" as soon as they are received.

All checks have standard information that is preprinted. This information includes the following:

- Name and address of the payer
- Telephone number of the payer
- American Bank Association (ABA) number
- Preprinted sequential number on each check
- Space to enter the full date
- Space to enter the amount of the check in numerals
- Space to enter the amount of the check in writing
- Space for the signature of the payer

- Space to enter the name of the payee, after the phrase "Pay to the order of"
- Preprinted name and address of bank
- Magnetic ink character recognition (MICR)

 Key Focus: An "ABA number" is located in the lower-left corner of a printed check. It is a nine-digit number that identifies the bank in which the checking account exists.

Key Focus: "MICR" is a character-recognition technology that is used in banking. A line of numbers is used on the bottom of checks and deposit slips for identification; this line can be read by automatic devices.

Deposits

Checks or cash should be deposited into a bank account promptly for the following reasons:

- They may be lost, misplaced, or stolen
- There is the possibility of a stop-payment order
- They may have a restricted time for cashing

Key Focus: Check or cash deposits must always be verified against bank statements that are received.

Key Focus: Besides accepting checks, patients may pay in cash, by debit or credit card, and via online payment systems.

Scheduling Bill Payments

A schedule for paying monthly expenses can be established in the accounting software, and includes

- Medical and office supplies
- Utilities
- Rent or mortgage
- Insurance premiums
- Taxes
- Postage
- Equipment rental
- Waste removal
- Housekeeping
- Laundry

STANDARD BILLING PROCEDURES

Most medical offices receive payments from insurance carriers, and then bill patients for any balances that are due.

Preparing Statements

All statements must include the following:

- Physician's name, address, phone number
- Patient's name and address
- Guarantor's name (if different from the patient)
- Balance from the previous month
- Itemized list: services, charges; by date, for current month
- Payments from patient or insurer during the month
- Total balance due

STANDARD COLLECTION PROCEDURES

Many patients pay their balance after each visit, and some pay within a standard 30-day period. However, some patients do not pay even after 30 days. Specific laws that are related to collection of payment include

- Statutes of limitations—state laws that set time limits for collection:
  - Open-book account—left open to charges made on an intermittent basis
  - Written-contract account—the practitioner and patient sign an agreement regarding treatments and payments
  - Single-entry account—consists of only one charge

Collection techniques that may be used include

- Initial telephone calls—begin 30 to 45 days after payment has not been received
- Follow-up statements and collection letters—begin 60 days after payment has not been received

Chapter 8
Health Insurance

HEALTH INSURANCE

Health insurance is a written contract, such as a policy or certificate of coverage, between a policyholder and an insurance company.

Basic Insurance Terminology

Health insurance is also known as medical insurance, and utilizes certain basic terminology. A *policyholder* is also called the *insured*, the *member*, or the *subscriber*. Important terms include

- Premium—an amount (usually monthly) paid by a policyholder to the insurance company
- Benefits—payments for services, by an insurance company, for a specified time period
- Lifetime maximum benefit—a total sum paid by a health plan over a patient's lifetime
- Dependents—spouses or children of policyholders
- First party—the patient (policyholder)
- Second party—the licensed practitioner who provides medical services
- Third party—the insurance company that carries risks of paying for healthcare services (*third-party payer*)
- Implied contract—when patient seeks healthcare services and practitioner agrees to treat patient, a financial contract is signed by patient assuming legal responsibility to pay; costs not covered by third-party insurer are the responsibility of the patient

- Deductible—a fixed dollar amount required to be paid by (also known as "met" by) the insured for provider charges, once per year in addition to the premium, prior to the third-party payer beginning to cover expenses
- Coinsurance—a fixed percentage of covered charges after deductible is met; rate is the health plan's percentage of the charge, followed by insured's percentage (often, 80% by insurance company and 20% by insured)
- Copayment—a fixed fee collected at the time of a patient visit; it is used in managed care plans such as health maintenance organizations (HMOs), instead of paying coinsurance
- Preferred provider—the practitioner preferred by an insurance plan to treat the patient
  - The plan pays this practitioner a set "contracted rate," agreed on for each service
  - The practitioner then accepts payment, with the patient's copayment as *payment in full*
  - Any remaining balance is adjusted off the patient's account to bring the balance to zero
- Exclusions—certain expenses that are not covered under the insured's contract
- Formulary—list of approved medications; plans often require use of medications listed on plan's formulary; substitutions may be allowed, with additional charges, or not allowed
- Elective procedure—planned procedures, done at convenience of the provider and patient; often covered by third-party payers, but only if certain rules are followed prior to the procedures
- Precertification—the process of confirming, with the insurance company, that the plan offers coverage for a certain procedure or service; some offices perform a preauthorization (prior authorization) as well

- Covered service—a proposed procedure or service for a patient that is required to be performed
- Medically necessary—a procedure or service that the insurance carrier agrees is required for a patient; a prior authorization number will be issued that approves the need for the procedure or service; however, this does not mean that the carrier agrees to pay for the service
- Predetermination—the carrier informs the provider of the maximum amount paid for a medically necessary service; then, documentation about the procedure or service must match the procedure codes submitted to the carrier, or the charges may be denied by the carrier

GOVERNMENT PLANS

Medicare

Medicare provides insurance for U.S. citizens aged 65 and older, dependent widows aged 50–65, the disabled and blind persons, workers of any age with chronic kidney disease requiring dialysis or end-stage renal disease requiring transplant, and kidney donors. There are four parts of Medicare:

- Part A—hospital insurance benefits, financed by Federal Insurance Contributions Act (FICA) tax on income
- Part B—covers (usually) 80% of allowed charges for many outpatient procedures and supplies
- Part C—provides choices called Medicare Advantage plans (PPOs, HMOs, private fee-for-service plans, special needs plans, and Medicare medical savings account plans)
- Part D—the prescription drug plan; offered by private insurance companies through contracts with Medicare; it provides limited benefits for prescription drugs

Medicare Plan Options

Medicare plan options include the original version (fee-for-service) and Medicare Advantage plans, which offer different types of managed care.

- Fee-for-service—allows choice of any licensed practitioner certified by Medicare. Fees are billed every time outpatient services are received; part of the fees is covered by Medicare and part by beneficiary.
  - Once annual deductible is met, Medicare pays 80% of approved charges directly to provider.
  - The patient pays the remaining 20% and any disallowed charges.
- Managed care plans—charge monthly premium, small copayment for office visits, but no deductible. Usually, an approved primary care provider (PCP) must be seen. They cover physical examinations and immunizations.

  - Preferred provider organizations (PPOs)—have networks of providers, hospitals that provide insurance companies or employers with services for members or employees at discounted rates.
    - Patients select a PCP, receive referrals for care outside network; PPOs are usually more expensive than traditional HMOs but less expensive than older fee-for-service plans
  - Private fee-for-service plans—patients choose from approved providers or facilities. Private insurers operate these plans, and determine rates. Physicians can bill for amounts not covered by these plans. Copayments may or may not be required.
  - Recovery audit contractor (RAC) program—designed to reduce Medicare fraud. Four different RACs monitor overpayments and underpayments in different parts of the country.

> 🩺 **Key Focus:** Medigap is a private insurance policy that supplements Medicare coverage to fill "gaps" in Part A and Part B coverage.

> 🩺 **Key Focus:** One of the important aspects in Medicare billing is the form called the *advance beneficiary notice (ABN)* or *waiver*.

Table 8-1 lists the advantages and disadvantages of managed care organizations (MCOs).

> 🩺 **Key Focus:** Managed care organizations (*managed care plans*) are not a separate type of insurance, but a way of offering services to patients enrolled in a group health plan, self-insured plan, or individual health plan.

Medicaid

It covers low-income, blind, or disabled patients; needy families; foster children; and children born with birth defects.

- It is a health cost assistance program, and not an insurance program.
- Government provides assistance to recipients, patients at no charge; subscribers, patients pay for insurance programs through premiums.
- The government provides funds to every state to cover specified, mandated services. Each state then adds its own funds for additional optional services, such as

    - Early diagnostic screening/treatment for age 21 or less
    - Emergency services

Table 8-1 *Advantages and Disadvantages of Managed Care*

Advantages	Disadvantages
Smaller out-of-pocket patient expenses	Increase paperwork
Nominal copayments paid by patients	Preauthorization is required
No deduction in certain plans	Reimbursement rates are lower
Healthcare costs contained	Physician choices are limited
Authorized services are paid for	Coverage may not be renewed
Establishment of fee schedules	Occasional limits on specialized care
Usually cover preventative medical treatment	Occasional limits on referrals
	Limits on flexibility
	Nonauthorized or nonapproved treatments are not covered

- Laboratory services and x-rays
- Licensed, credentialed practitioner services
- Skilled nursing facility (SNF) care
- Child vaccines.

Accepting Assignment

Licensed practitioners treating Medicaid patients agree to accept established Medicaid payments as *payment in full*.

This is called *accepting assignment*. For services *not* covered, providers bill patients directly. If the patient has private insurance, it must be billed first.

Dual Coverage
Elderly or disabled Medicare patients who cannot pay differences between charges and Medicare payments may also qualify for Medicaid. Balances are not billed unless a noncovered service is provided and the patient is notified, or the balance is determined to be billable.

State Guidelines
Medicaid benefits vary between states, with eligibility based on reported monthly income. Guidelines are as follows:

- Do not submit claims without verification of benefit eligibility
- Ensure that providers sign all claims unless they are electronically submitted
- Send claims to state's approved contractor
- Except for emergencies, authorization is often required before performing services
- Check deadlines for claim submission with the state Medicaid office
- Medicaid patients must be treated professionally and with courtesy

TRICARE and CHAMPVA

TRICARE (for the military, replaced the program known as CHAMPUS)—for families of uniformed personnel and retirees; it offers three plans, each with different types of benefits:

- TRICARE Standard (fee-for-service)
- TRICARE Prime (an HMO)
- TRICARE Extra (a PPO)

CHAMPVA—Civilian Health and Medical Program of the Veterans Administration; it covers dependent spouses and children of veterans with total, permanent, service-connected disabilities.

- Also covers surviving spouses and dependent children of veterans who died in the line of duty or from service-connected disabilities

TRICARE and CHAMPVA Eligibility

TRICARE enrollees must have valid identification cards, and be enrolled in the computerized Defense Enrollment Eligibility Reporting System (DEERS). CHAMPVA eligibility is determined by Veterans Affairs medical centers.

State Children's Health Insurance Plan (CHIP)

State Children's Health Insurance Plan—commonly known as CHIP, it covers uninsured children in families with incomes too high to qualify for Medicaid, but too low to afford private insurance.

Affordable Care Act

It created state-based American Health Benefit Exchanges through which individuals can purchase coverage.

- Premium and cost-sharing credits available if income is between 133% and 400% of federal poverty level; it also created exchanges through which small businesses can purchase coverage.
- This Act expanded Medicaid coverage to millions of low-income Americans and attempted to improve both Medicaid and CHIP. Also extended funding for CHIP.
- It created a minimum Medicaid income eligibility level across the United States.

- Those newly eligible for Medicaid received equivalent benefits that included the minimum essential benefits provided by the Affordable Insurance Exchanges.

Medical assistants help patients understand their policies and determine the type of coverage they have. Table 8-2 lists types of service coverage.

> **Key Focus:** Some patients have prescription drug coverage. It is an add-on plan to a main insurance policy, and sometimes has a separate deductible and different copayment.

Health Insurance

PRIVATE HEALTH PLANS

Medical assistants must understand private health plans' rules and regulations in order to explain information to providers and patients. Most Americans are covered by group policies, usually through their employers.

Fee Schedules and Changes

Physicians establish their own *usual fees* for frequently performed procedures and services. These are listed in *fee schedules*. Examples include *initial office visit*, *follow-up visit*, *consultations*, *hospital admission or consultation*, *emergency room visit*, and various types of tests.

Fee-for-Service and Managed Care Plans

The two major types of health plans are *traditional fee-for-service plans* and *managed care plans*.

- Fee-for-service plans—oldest and most expensive type. They pay practitioners a set amount for each service,

Table 8-2 *Types of Service Coverage*

Type of Coverage	Description
Ancillary	Supplemental riders for alternative, dental, and vision care as well as prescription drugs
Catastrophic care	Emergency protection against only high-cost, unexpected medical services. All routine and sick care is paid for out of pocket
Disease-specific	Supplemental insurance for specific chronic or terminal illnesses (Alzheimer's disease, cancer, heart disease, kidney failure, multiple sclerosis, Parkinson's disease, stroke)
Hospital services	Inpatient hospital care including room and board; also, facility fees for special services, including laboratory, operating room, and radiology
Physician services	Physician's fees for hospital or office visits, and nonsurgical procedures
Preventive care	Annual preventive care examinations, screening tests, and immunizations
Surgical services	Surgeon, anesthesiologist fees for surgery in a hospital, physician's office, outpatient surgical center

Health Insurance

based on a fee schedule listed in the policy. The patient is responsible for the balance.

- Managed care plans —managed care organizations enroll policyholders and providers. Services are provided at reduced rates. Enrolled providers are called *participating providers*. They are paid either by contracted fees or via capitation. Examples include
  - Preferred provider organizations
  - Health maintenance organizations—require members to choose a *PCP* ("gatekeeper"), who oversees their care, makes referrals to specialists, and approves additional services if needed. Wellness and preventive medicine are emphasized.

There are many types of HMOs, which include

- Group-model HMOs—multispecialty practices; may be reimbursed via capitation; less common today due to prevalence of fee-for-service plans
- Staff-model HMOs—employ providers; all services provided by the practice; emergency care needs no preauthorization; PCP handles routine care and referrals
- Exclusive provider organizations (EPOs)—patients use the plan's provider network exclusively; PCPs not required; specialist referrals not needed; preauthorization required for expensive services; usually less expensive than PPOs
- Independent practice associations (IPAs)—managed care organizations that consist of providers practicing in their own individual offices; they provide better leverage in establishing contracts with HMOs and other insurers
- Point-of-service (POS) plans—allow more freedom in choice of care; PCPs are not required and patients can see specialists without referrals; choosing

providers who are part of these plans is less expensive

Commercial Payers

Commercial health insurance plans—from private companies that control premium prices and types of benefits. Examples include Blue Cross Blue Shield Association, which offers many varieties of plans.

Blue Cross Blue Shield Association
Blue Cross Blue Shield Association is a nationwide federation of nonprofit and for-profit service organizations. They provide prepaid healthcare services to subscribers. Plans vary widely between individual states and individual plans.

Private Commercial Carriers
There are many differences between private commercial carriers. Examples include
- Liability insurance—also called *personal injury insurance*. It covers injuries caused by the insured or that occurred on the insured's property. Individuals or companies may purchase liability insurance.
- Disability insurance—covers people injured or disabled for non-work-related reasons. It may be either offered by employees for free or paid for by employees. It can also be purchased by self-employed individuals. It does not cover medical expenses.

Health Insurance

> **Key Focus:** Workers' compensation is private insurance that covers employment-related accidents and diseases, generally covered by third-party liability insurance.

Patient-Centered Medical Home

A patient-centered medical home, or *primary care medical home*, offers the following:

- Accessible service—shorter wait times, more "in person" office hours, unlimited access to providers via telephone and computer, e-mail, and telemedicine
- Comprehensive care—preventive care and wellness, acute and chronic, traditional medical facilities as well as virtual links to patient care within the community
- Coordinated care—includes hospitals, specialty care, community services, home healthcare, and other support; it is very important before, during, and after hospital discharge
- Patient-centered care—primary care focused on the whole person; providers partner with patients and their families, considering individual culture, needs, preferences, and values
- Safety and quality—evidence-based medicine, clinical decision support tools, monitoring patient experiences and satisfaction, and public sharing of safety and data improvement activities

PAYER PAYMENT SYSTEMS

Many payers reimburse using fee schedules. Others such as Medicare use formulas and processes.

Medicare Payment System: RBRVS

The Medicare payment system—the *resource-based relative value scale (RBRVS)* establishes relative value units, replacing usual or historical charges with amounts based on what each service actually costs to provide (often less than each physician's fee schedule).

- RBRVS fees have three parts, multiplied together, as follows:
  - The national uniform *relative value unit (RVU)*—based on the physician's work, overhead, and the cost of malpractice insurance
  - A *geographic adjustment factor (GAF)*—used to adjust the relative value units to reflect the relative costs, such as the practice's rent and utilities, based on geographic area
  - A nationally uniform *conversion factor (CF)*—an amount used as a multiplier to adjust charges based on the *cost-of-living index*

Payment Methods

Most third-party payers use one of three common methods to reimburse providers. These include allowed charges, a contracted fee schedule, and capitation.

Allowed Charges
Allowed charges are maximum amounts a payer will pay any provider for each procedure or service. They are also called *maximum allowable fees*, *maximum charges*, *allowed amounts*, *allowed fees*, and *allowable charges.*

Contracted Fee Schedule
A contracted fee schedule is often used by payers such as PPOs, and establishes fixed fee schedules with physicians.

It determines percentages of charges paid by the payer as well as the patient. Participating providers bill patients usual charges for services not covered by the plan.

Capitation

Capitation is defined as a fixed prepayment for each member and is determined by a managed care plan that initiates contracts with healthcare providers. It may cover preventive care, counseling, telephone calls, office visits, injections, immunizations, tests, and many medical treatments.

Various types of health insurance plans that offer different levels of coverage for various prices are shown in Figure 8-1.

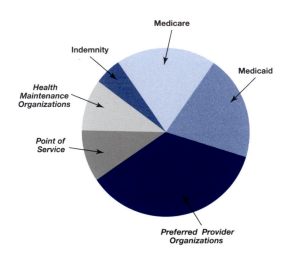

Figure 8-1 *Types of Insurance Payers.*

THE CLAIMS PROCESS

The process of health insurance claims requires a variety of steps to be performed.

Obtaining Patient Information

Patient information is usually filled in on a patient registration form.

Basic Facts

- Patient name, home address and telephone number, date of birth, Social Security number
- Next of kin, or person to contact in case of emergency
- Insurance information, as follows:
  - Name of subscriber or insured
  - Signature of patient authorizing release of information to insurer
  - Signature of patient for assignment of benefits
  - Current employer, address, phone number
  - Insurance carrier, effective coverage date, group plan, and I.D. numbers

Eligibility for Services

- Copy or scan both sides of the patient's insurance card.
- Obtain release signatures and put them in the patient's financial record.
- Verify the effective date of insurance coverage.
- Inform patients in writing, before services are performed, that they may not be covered.
- Collect patients' signatures that signify their acceptance of responsibility to pay for noncovered services.
- Keep original waivers of liability in patients' financial records.
- Provide a copy of these waivers to patients.

Obtaining Authorization

- Call insurance companies or use their websites to receive prior authorization.
- Have all patient or subscriber information available, including procedure names, as well as CPT and ICD codes, when you contact insurers.
- Document all authorization information provided by the insurer.
- Authorization is given immediately or within 24 hours.
- Keep authorization information in the patient record.
- Authorization numbers will be inserted into block 23 of the CMS-1500 claim form.

Coordination of Benefits

This prevents payment duplication by restricting insurance company payments to no more than 100% of covered benefit costs. This includes policyholder deductibles, coinsurance, and copayments.

- The *primary plan* pays benefits first. It is always the employer group health plan.
- The *secondary* (supplemental) plan pays deductible and coinsurance or copayment.
- If, for example, husband and wife are covered by two or more medical plans, the *birthday rule* may be followed. It states that the insurance policy of the policyholder whose birthday comes first in the calendar year is the primary payer for all dependents.

Delivering Services to Patients

All services delivered to patients and referrals to outside licensed practitioners must be entered into patient record.

Practitioner Services

Licensed practitioners add patient symptoms, the diagnosis, the treatment plan, prescribed medications, and when a follow-up visit is needed to the medical record. Then, an encounter form (superbill) or charge slip is filled out, including the diagnosis, treatment, and, sometimes, the fee.

- The practitioner instructs patient to give this paperwork to medical assistant before leaving the office.
- If copayment is needed from the patient, it should be collected before or after seeing the practitioner.

Medical Coding

Most medical offices use superbills that are preprinted with common procedures and their codes. If charges are not preprinted, there is a space near each procedure where current charges can be inserted. Blank spaces at the bottom can be completed with needed information.

- Procedures checked off on these forms must have been completed—this is verified by comparing the superbill with the medical record. This protects against fraudulent charges.
- Appropriate diagnosis codes must be checked off to prove medical necessity.
- If a charge slip is used, medical assistant must translate listed procedures into charge codes for insurer.

Referrals and Authorizations for Other Services

Medical assistants may need to secure authorization from insurers for additional procedures to be provided outside their medical offices. These include hospital or ambulatory surgical center services. The insurer must be contacted and the reason for the procedure(s) explained.

- Authorization numbers must be obtained for the procedure(s). Numbers are entered into the billing program for inclusion on related claims.
- Medical assistant may have to arrange appointments for required services, especially if urgently needed.
- It should be verified with the insurer that the request specialist is approved. A referral may also be needed so that charges will be covered.

Preparing and Transmitting the Healthcare Claim

The following information should be included for all claims:

- Address of the insured
- Insured's identification number
- Name of the insured
- Name of the insured's insurance company
- Patient's information
- Patient's signature for releasing information needed for a claim form to be completed
- Telephone number of the insured
- Amount billed by the physician

Key Focus: The *review* determines amount of deductible or coinsurance that patient owes. The amount owed to the practice is called the *patient's liability*.

It is important to follow these tips when entering data in a medical billing program:

- Enter data only in capital letters
- Avoid using prefixes such as Mr., Ms., or Dr.

- Avoid hyphens, commas, apostrophes, and other special characters unless required to be used by the insurer
- Use only valid data in all fields, and avoid using words such as "SAME"
- Electronic claims include five major sections: provider, subscriber (insured or policyholder), patient (subscriber or another person), claim details, and services
- Taxonomy code—a 10-digit number that represents the provider's medical specialty

Transmitting Electronic Claims

All medical offices were mandated to be in compliance with electronic filing of claim forms, between computers, by October 2003. Electronic claim submissions require the same information that is part of the CMS-1500 form. As of 2015, all claims must be submitted electronically.

- The electronic claim form is called the *HIPAA Healthcare Claim or Equivalent Encounter Information (5010 claim or 837P claim).* Its official name is the *X12 837 Health Care Claim.*

Key Focus: Errors may also occur on electronic claims. Therefore, it is essential for the medical assistant to proofread all claims prior to submitting them.

To send a claim electronically, you must

- Collect all information needed about the patient
- Connect computer to insurance company's computer server, using instructions provided by insurer
- Fill out the claim form as you would fill out the CMS-1500

Key Focus: Software programs are available that allow claim processing without the need to re-enter some of the data more than once.

Paper Claim Completion

The CMS-1500 health insurance claim form is the most common form that is used for paper claims as well as for electronic claim submission. Its electronic form is called the *ANSI X12N 837P*. The CMS-1500 is also known as the *universal claim form.*

The claim form may be submitted to an insurance carrier or third-party payer via a paper claim form (mailing) or by electronic media claim (EMC).

Key Focus: Never use punctuation, decimals, dollar signs, or correction aids on claim forms. There should be no items taped, clipped, or stapled to claim forms.

The Role of the Medical Assistant Regarding Health Insurance Claims

Medical assistants are very important in the health insurance claims process. They must

- Answer patient's questions about this process, including how owed fees are determined.
- Regularly verify insurance coverage of patients, and often explain details of coverage to them.
- Be able to accurately prepare health insurance claims.
- Follow up on claims that are past due.
- Attempt to collect unpaid amounts.

- Be aware that their roles are different based on each type of medical practice.

Transmitting Claims Directly

Direct transmission of claims uses translators and communications technology, which helps *electronic data interchange (EDI)*.

Using Clearinghouses

A *clearinghouse* is a company that helps medical offices send and receive data in the correct EDI format. They are essential when the type of medical billing software used does not include translation software. Other services provided by clearinghouses include

- Translation of nonstandard formats into standard formats
- "Scrubbing claims"—to ensure that they meet coding and payer claim standards and will be paid quickly
- Checking of software for errors and missing information
- Ensuring that medical offices send out all required data elements

Using Direct Data Entry

Online *direct data entry (DDE)* allows standard data elements to be sent via the Internet. For this, EDI formatting is not required. Data are loaded directly in the computers of the health plan. However, every claim must be hand-keyed into the system every time the patient is seen.

Generating Clean Claims

To generate "clean" claims, which contain no errors, refer to the insurance company's most recent *claim submission manual*. The most common errors that occur are as follows:

- Missing Medicare assignment indicator or benefits assignment indicator
- Missing or incomplete service or billing provider information and identification
- Missing or invalid information about secondary insurance plans
- Missing or invalid patient or subscriber information, including misspelled names
- Missing parts of names or identifiers of referring providers
- Missing payer names or identifiers, which are required by all payers

Claims Security

For security of electronic claims, data must pass through a computer *firewall*, which examines them for any potentially harmful contents. Additional claims security measures include

- Access control, log files, and passwords—which keep intruders out
- Backups—saved copies of files that can replace items after computer damage occurs
- Security policies—steps taken to handle any violations that occur

Claim Form Rejection

The following factors are the most common reasons for claim rejection:

- Duplicate dates of service
- Incorrect place of service
- Missing/incorrect diagnosis code

- Missing/incorrect modifier
- Missing/incorrect referring physician
- Missing/incorrect number of days or units
- Missing/incorrect patient information (name, address, insurance number)
- Missing/invalid procedure code

Insurer Processing Claims

The Claims Register

Electronic claims are listed in a log of transmitted claims that allows them to be tracked. For paper claims, a *claims register* should be created that documents claims created in this manner. Insurers regularly review all transmitted claims, most of which is done electronically.

Review for Medical Necessity

Procedures/diagnoses are regularly reviewed by insurers to determine whether treatments are medically necessary.

Review for Allowable Benefits

Claims departments also compare providers' charged fees with patients' health insurance policy benefits. This is done to determine the amount of deductible or coinsurance owed by the patient. The amount owed by the patient is known as the *patient liability*.

Payment and Remittance Advice

When the insurer accepts a claim, a benefit is then paid to the provider or the patient. This depends on whether an *assignment of benefits* was signed, as well as on the insurance policy. The insurer also sends a *remittance advice*, which is an explanation of payment or benefits.

- The remittance advice may be electronic or printed
- Every insurance plan has its own remittance advice format

Health Insurance

- When multiple patients are listed on the remittance advice, it is important to mark out all information that should not be seen by any unauthorized person
- The remittance advice includes the following information:
  - Name of insured, I.D. number, patient name
  - Claim number
  - Date and place of service, procedure code for provided service
  - Amount billed by provider, amount allowed
  - Amount of patient liability (coinsurance, copayment, deductible, noncovered services)
  - Amount paid
  - Notation of noncovered services, with explanation of reason

Billing and Reimbursement Cycle

The billing and reimbursement cycle includes 10 steps:

- Collection of patient information
- Verification of insurance
- Preparation of encounter forms
- Coding (diagnoses and procedures)
- Review of linkage and compliance
- Calculation of physician charges
- Preparation of claims
- Transmission of claims
- Adjudication of payers
- Follow-up of reimbursements and retention of records

Key Focus: Filing timelines mean most insurance carriers accept claims up to 1 year from the date of service. Some have timelines as short as 90 days.

HEALTH INSURANCE PORTABILITY AND ACCOUNTABILITY ACT (HIPAA)

This Act was passed to address many problems concerning health insurance. Its privacy, security, and breach notification rules protect privacy and security of health information. They also provide individuals with certain rights to their own health information.

Protected Health Information

Covered entities must

- Adopt a set of privacy practices
- Appoint a staff member as privacy official for ensuring privacy practices are adopted and followed
- Notify patients about their privacy rights
- Secure patient records of individually identifiable health information so that they are not available to those who do not need them
- Train employees on privacy practices

Key Focus: HIPAA is very specific concerning confidentiality. Fines may be up to $250,000 per incident, or jail up to 10 years for violation of HIPAA laws.

Privacy Rule

The HIPAA privacy rule covers the use and disclosure of patients' protected health information (PHI), including

- Patient name and address
- Account number
- Birth date
- E-mail address, fax number
- Health plan beneficiary number

- Social Security number
- Telephone numbers
- Photographic images
- Physical description to identify patient

PREAUTHORIZATION

Preauthorization from health insurance providers may be required for certain services. Preauthorization (precertification or required prior approval) requires

- The patient's medical record and insurance information
- A precertification form
- Specific service or procedure requested, along with number of treatments, period of time to complete them
- Specific physician documentation in the patient's record that supports the requested service or procedure
- Name, address, phone and fax number of provider who will perform requested service or procedure

Key Focus: Preauthorization is usually obtained a minimum of 24 hours before a patient arrives for an office visit, hospitalization, or a certain procedure or treatment.

CHAPTER 9
Diagnostic and Procedural Coding

Medical assistants must be familiar with medical coding, to correctly generate healthcare claims. *Diagnostic coding* represents diagnoses given to patients by physicians, while *procedure coding* represents services provided.

DIAGNOSTIC CODING

Each patient's diagnoses are submitted to insurance carriers as specific codes during the claims process. Numeric and alphanumeric codes are used. They are known as ICD (International Classification of Diseases) codes. The newest edition of these codes is the ICD-10-CM, which became effective October 1, 2015. It is the 10th edition.

Why Diagnosis Codes Are Used

Diagnosis codes contain

- The patient's chief complaint (CC)
- The practitioner's established diagnosis (Dx)
- Any coexisting conditions (comorbidities)

This information should prove medical necessity for treatments provided. ICD codes are based on the United Nations' *World Health Organization (WHO)* system. Diagnosis codes are updated every year on October 1, while procedural codes are updated on January 1.

Key Focus: The edition of diagnosis codes being used is based on the date of service (DOS)—not on the date that a claim is submitted.

ICD-10-CM codes are used for the following:

- Facilitating payment for services
- Evaluating patterns of how patients use healthcare facilities
- Studying healthcare costs
- Researching healthcare quality
- Predicting healthcare trends
- Planning for future health-related needs

ICD-10-CM INFORMATION

The *International Classification of Diseases, Tenth Revision, Clinical Modification* is abbreviated as "ICD-10-CM." It lists diseases and injuries with codes of up to seven digits. It is a major revision of the ICD-9-CM. Though similar in design, the actual codes used are very different, and there are 21 instead of 17 chapters.

Key Focus: First three digits of ICD-10 codes are called the *category* or *rubric*, followed by decimal point. If conditions exist that help specify the three-digit code, up to four additional digits may be added. A *placeholder* character (like "X") is used after the fourth digit.

Key Focus: Assigning codes must be done carefully for accuracy in claims, within the scope of practice.

Comparisons Between ICD-9-CM and ICD-10-CM

The ICD-10-CM allows for increased specificity for diagnosis classifications. It provides expansion for new codes. This is vital when linking diagnosis and CPT procedure codes to prove medical necessity. The basic comparisons between ICD-9-CM and ICD-10-CM are shown in Table 9-1.

Table 9-1 *Comparing ICD-9-CM and ICD-10-CM*

ICD-9-CM	ICD-10-CM
14,200 codes	More than 68,000 codes
3–5 characters (first is alpha or numeric, others are numeric)	3–7 characters (first is uppercase alpha, 2–3 are numeric, and 4–7 are alpha or numeric)
Specificity is limited	Specificity is expanded
No laterality (meaning "side of the body affected")	Has laterality, indicating side of the body affected
Decimal points not always used after third character	Decimal point must be used after third character
Placeholder "zero" as fourth digit is present when a fifth digit is required	A placeholder "X" is used for a nonexistent digit when a sixth or seventh digit is needed for code specificity
Some combination codes are used	An expanded number of combination codes are used
External causes of morbidity and mortality, including poisonings, are listed as "E codes"	Instead of a separate code section, external causes are listed as V01–Y99 codes
Factors influencing health status are listed as "V codes"	Instead of a separate code section, health status codes are listed as Z00–Z99 codes

Diagnostic

Alphabetic and Numeric Indexes

Both the ICD-9-CM and ICD-10-CM have an *alphabetic index* of diseases, conditions, and terms. It is located in the front of the book. Once the correct diagnostic term is found, you use lists of appropriate codes found in the *Tabular List*, which contains the 21 chapters. A *category* or *rubric* has three characters; a *subcategory* has four characters.

Characters and Specificity

All ICD-10 codes begin with an alpha character and may be up to seven characters in total. While *breast cancer* was identified in the ICD-9 as the code *233.0* (carcinoma in situ breast), the ICD-10 identifies it as

- *D05.01* (lobular carcinoma in situ of right breast)
- *D05.02* (lobular carcinoma in situ of left breast)
- *D05.11* (intraductal carcinoma in situ of right breast)
- *D05.12* (intraductal carcinoma in situ of left breast)

You can see the increased specificity of the ICD-10-CM in this example.

Placeholders

The ICD-10 uses an "X" as a placeholder for future expansion of a code's specificity. For example, when a scalp abrasion occurs, the code is *S00.01*, but there is a note to check for three options indicated by "check X7th." The code is listed as S00.01X, followed by one of three letters A, D, or S, as follows:

- S00.01XA—abrasion of scalp, initial encounter
- S00.01XD—abrasion of scalp, subsequent encounter
- S00.01XS—abrasion of scalp, sequela (pathological condition resulting from this injury)

Combination Codes

A combination code describes two diagnoses within one code. It often describes a diagnosis with an associated *manifestation*, or *secondary process.* The ICD-10 has many of these, reducing the need for multiple codes for more complicated diagnoses. An example is R65.21, which describes "severe sepsis with septic shock."

An Overview of ICD-10-CM

The ICD-10-CM coding manual contains two volumes of information, including

- Volume I—Tabular List
  - Twenty-one chapters of disease and injury codes, organized by etiology or body system
  - Supplementary classification, found in each chapter
  - Codes are arranged in numerical order
  - *Note:* The E and V codes used in the ICD-9-CM have been removed
- Volume II—Alphabetic Index
  - First part: diseases and injures
  - Second part: external causes
  - Tables of neoplasms, drugs, chemicals
  - Lists main terms in alphabetical order, with indented subterms under the main terms

Conventions

Conventions are items that provide basic guidelines for coding. They include a list of abbreviations, punctuation,

Diagnostic

symbols, typefaces, and instructional notes, appearing at the beginning of the ICD-10. Examples are as follows:

- INCLUDES—entries following this word define the preceding entry to a larger degree.
- EXCLUDES1—the code is excluded and never should be used at the same time as the code above this term.
- EXCLUDES2—"not included here"; the excluded condition is not part of the condition represented by the code; however, if documented, both conditions may be present at the same time.
- Use additional code—indicates an additional code should be used if available, after the primary code.
- Code first underlying disease—this appears when the category is not to be used as the primary diagnosis.
- Code first, if applicable, any causal condition—the code may be used as a primary diagnosis if the causal condition is unknown or not applicable.
- *See* Condition—refers to a different "main term" for the condition.
- *See also*—a suggestion that a better code may be found elsewhere for the diagnosis being coded.
- Brackets ([ ]) in the Tabular List indicate synonyms, alternative wordings, or explanations; in the Alphabetic Index, they indicate that two codes are required. The code in the bracket is the *secondary code*.
- Colons (:) are used in the Tabular List after an incomplete term that needs one of the terms that follow to make it assignable to a given category.
- NEC—"not elsewhere classified" is used when ICD-10 does not have a code specific enough for condition.
- NOS—"not otherwise specified" or "unspecified." In general, codes with NOS should be avoided.
- Parentheses () are used around descriptions that do not affect the code.

The Alphabetic Index

This contains all medical terms necessary to locate codes in the Tabular List, organized by condition. Search first for the condition (e.g., fracture) and then location (ankle). Main terms are printed in boldface type, followed by their code numbers. Any listed subterms may show disease causes, or describe body sites or related types of information.

The Tabular List

This consists of the 21 chapters of disease descriptions and codes. All body systems are covered, and other chapters cover injuries related to poisonings, anaphylactic reactions, and external causes. There is also a chapter on health encounters for healthy patients, including physicals and well-child visits. Coding rules include the following:

- Codes containing four to seven characters must be reported on claims since they represent the most specific diagnosis on the patient's medical record.
  - This is called *coding to the highest level of specificity*.
- Decimal points are used after the third character of a code but are never placed on claim forms.

Coding with the ICD-10-CM

Every diagnosis and procedure that is selected on an encounter form is required to be verified in the medical record. Often, the most specific diagnosis code for a patient's condition is not listed on the encounter form, and you may be required to find the most appropriate code. The following additional guidelines are also followed:

- Acute or subacute conditions (having sudden onset), or chronic conditions that suddenly worsen.
- Chronic conditions are those that have persisted for a longer time.

- When available, combination codes are used instead of two single codes, for more complicated diagnoses.
- However, there are times when more than one code is needed to fully explain a condition.

Additional Guidelines for ICD-10 Coding
The following guidelines help to make coding procedures more efficient and specific:

- Acute versus chronic conditions—acute as well as subacute conditions are those of sudden onset, or chronic conditions that have suddenly become worse.
  - Some conditions, such as bronchitis, cause the patient to have both the acute form (J20.9) and the underlying chronic form (J42).
  - When two codes must be reported, acute code is listed first, followed by chronic code.
- Combination codes—when available, they must be used in place of the two single codes.
  - Example: If patient has cholelithiasis (gallstones) as well as acute cholecystitis (gallbladder inflammation), the combination code K80.10 is used instead of two separate codes.
- Multiple coding—before the ICD-10, codes often did not fully describe a diagnosis. This happens less often now because of the ICD-10's better, more complete codes.

  - However, more than one code is sometimes needed to completely explain a diagnosis.
  - Example: When a disease or condition manifests or results from another disease or condition.

Coding Unclear Diagnoses
When diagnoses are unclear, symptoms that resulted in the patient seeking care should be used for coding, until an absolute diagnosis is made. This is true for *outpatient coding*,

but not for *inpatient coding*. For impending or threatened conditions, check to see whether there is an existing code. If not, code the underlying symptoms or conditions.

Key Focus: ICD-10 codes always begin with a letter. Remember that in Chapter 15 (Pregnancy, Childbirth, and the Puerperium), first character is an "O", not "zero".

Principal Versus Primary Diagnosis

According to the *Uniform Hospital Discharge Data Set* or *UHDDS*, a "principal diagnosis" is the "condition established after study to be chiefly responsible for occasioning the admission of the patient to the hospital for care."

- Outpatient coding uses *primary diagnosis* instead of *principal diagnosis*, since it is the main reason for the patient's visit.
- The *secondary (subsequent) diagnosis* includes other conditions affecting the patient during the visit. They are coded after the primary diagnosis.

Diagnosis-Related Group and Inpatient (IP) Coding

Inpatient claims are paid based on a system called *diagnosis-related groups* or *DRGs*. More than 700 DRGs exist, based on principal diagnosis; other diagnoses; significant procedures performed; and the patient's age, sex, and discharge status. For correct coding, all information must be thorough and accurate.

External Cause of Injury and Health Status Codes

In the ICD-9, there were two extra chapters, "E codes" (for external causes) and "V codes" (for other factors influencing the patient seeking treatment). The ICD-10 incorporated the E codes and V codes into these chapters:

- Chapter 19—Injury, Poisoning, and Certain Other Consequences of External Causes: begin with "S" or "T"
- Chapter 20—External Causes of Morbidity: begin with "V", "W", "X", or "Y"
- Chapter 21—Supplementary Classification of Factors Influencing Health Status and Contact with Health Services: begin with "Z"

Health Status Codes
The "Z codes" in Chapter 21 are generally used in the outpatient setting, since patients are basically healthy:

- Z23—(encounter for) vaccination, which is a diagnosis code
- Z37.0—vaginal delivery of single, live-born newborn (status of newborn, for the mother's medical record)
- Z51.11—(encounter for) chemotherapy treatment
- Z88.0—history (personal) of allergy to penicillin

Z codes use the same Alphabetic Index for their coding. However, in the examples above, the terms *vaccination*, *encounter*, *history*, and *outcome of delivery* would be italicized in the Alphabetic Index.

External Cause Codes
The external cause codes that begin with "T", "V", and "Y" can be complicated. They are related to occurrences such as accidents, poisonings, falls, fires, environmental factors, assaults, and self-injury. Generally, external cause codes are only used for initial treatment for an acute condition, not subsequent visits—except for acute fractures.

Guidelines for their use include the following:

- Use as many external cause codes as needed to completely explain how the incident occurred.
- Use the correct *place of occurrence* code, found under the key term "place."
- If machinery or a motorized vehicle was involved, there will be a related code for its type.
- Often, the fourth character describes the person who was injured.
- A seventh character may be used to describe the type of counter ("A", "D", or "S").
- Placeholders such as the letter "X" are commonly used when needed.
- Poisonings and their adverse effects have six designations: *poisoning*, *accident*, *therapeutic use*, *suicide attempt*, *assault*, and *undetermined*. Often, combination codes are used for poisonings.
- Burns usually require three codes—the degree of the burn, the percentage of the body burned, and the external cause code for how the burn occurred.

Synopsis of ICD-10-CM Coding Guidelines, Chapter by Chapter

Table 9-2 lists chapters, descriptions, and code ranges for the ICD-10-CM.

PROCEDURAL CODING CPT

Current Procedural Terminology (CPT) is an important part of medical billing and reimbursement. Transferring a narrative description of procedures into numbers is called *procedural coding*. Five-digit procedure codes, in the CPT manual, from the American Medical Association are primarily used in hospitals and similar facilities.

Table 9-2 *ICD-10-CM Codes*

Chapter	Description	Code Range
1	Certain infectious and parasitic diseases	A00–B99
2	Neoplasms	C00–D49
3	Diseases of the blood and blood-forming organs, and certain disorders involving the immune mechanism	D50–D89
4	Endocrine, nutritional, and metabolic diseases	E00–E89
5	Mental and behavioral disorders	F01–F99
6	Diseases of the nervous system	G00–G99
7	Diseases of the eye and adnexa (accessory organs)	H00–H59
8	Diseases of the ear and mastoid process	H60–H95
9	Diseases of the circulatory system	I00–I99
10	Diseases of the respiratory system	J00–J99
11	Diseases of the digestive system	K00–K95
12	Diseases of the skin and subcutaneous tissue	L00–L99

Diagnostic

Table 9-2 (*Continued*)

Chapter	Description	Code Range
13	Diseases of the musculoskeletal system and connective tissue	M00–M99
14	Diseases of the genitourinary system	N00–N99
15	Pregnancy, childbirth, and the puerperium (the period of about 6 weeks after childbirth)	O00–O9A
16	Certain conditions originating in the perinatal period	P00–P96
17	Congenital malformations, deformations, and chromosomal abnormalities	Q00–Q99
18	Symptoms, signs, and abnormal clinical and laboratory findings; not elsewhere classified	R00–R99
19	Injury, poisoning, certain other consequences of external causes	S00–T88
20	External causes of morbidity	V00–Y99
21	Factors influencing health status and contact with health services	Z00–Z99

Diagnostic

Organization of the CPT Manual

There are six main sections of CPT codes. Except for the evaluation and management (E/M) codes, the sections are listed numerically, by code range. Since the evaluation and management codes are used so often, they were placed at the front of the manual for easy use. Table 9-3 lists CPT code ranges.

Sections of the CPT are divided into categories, which are then divided into headings based on types of tests, services, or body systems. Code number ranges are listed in the upper-right corner so that codes can be quickly located after using the index. Each page of the CPT lists other information, which includes

- The section name, which denotes each chapter
- The subsection name, which details the related body system

Table 9-3 *CPT Codes*

Section	Range of Codes
Evaluation and management	99201–99499
Anesthesiology	00100–01999, 99100–99140
Surgery	10021–69990
Radiology	70010–79999
Pathology and laboratory	80047–89398
Medicine (except anesthesia)	90281–99199, 99500–99607

- The subheading, which describes the body area within the body system
- The category, which describes the area of the procedure

General CPT Guidelines

Each CPT section has its own section guidelines, which include code format and add-on codes.

CPT Code Format

The majority of CPT codes have their complete description listed next to them. They are considered to be "standard codes." A difference occurs when a code description has a *semicolon*, which is followed by a code with an indented description—this means you must refer back to the previous code description to fully understand its meaning.

Example:

25500	Closed treatment of radial shaft fracture; without manipulation
25505	with manipulation

Read code 25500 up to the semicolon; then substitute the description for 25505 after the semicolon. This means that the full description for 25505 would be as follows: "Closed treatment of radial shaft fracture; with manipulation."

Add-On Codes

Add-on codes are used to describe procedures performed in addition to a primary procedure. A plus sign (+) is used to indicate add-on codes. Appendix D of the CPT manual contains a complete list of all add-on codes used. Add-on codes always follow a primary code and are never used alone.

Diagnostic

Symbols Used in CPT

Symbols commonly used in the CPT include

- A *red dot* or *bullet point* (•), which indicates a new procedure code
- *Facing triangles* (►◄), which indicate new or revised text
- A *blue triangle* (▲), which indicates revised code; this can influence the related procedure code
- An *arrow* (→), which signifies "Reference to CPT Assistant, CPT Changes" book
- A *circle with a diagonal line* (Ø), which indicates exemptions to modifier 51; this modifier is used when multiple procedures are performed in the same session; Appendix E lists all modifier 51 exempt codes
- An *asterisk* (*), which indicates a surgical procedure only
- The *# (pound) sign*, which denotes codes that are out of numeric sequence
- A *lightning bolt*, which denotes vaccines awaiting FDA approval; these vaccines are listed in Appendix K
- A *bull's eye*, which is a dot within a circle, denotes moderate, conscious sedation required for a procedure; this sedation is included as part of the procedure and cannot be billed separately

Modifiers

Modifiers indicate that a procedure may be reported using an "unlisted procedure" code, or by use of a modifier, which is a two-digit code preceded by a hyphen, clarifying the procedure. Modifiers are used primarily when

- A service or procedure was performed more than once, or by more than one physician.
- A service or procedure was increased or reduced.
- A procedure has two parts—a technical component and a professional component.

- Only part of a procedure was performed.
- A bilateral or multiple procedure was performed.
- Unusual difficulties occurred during the procedure.

> **Key Focus:** Up to four modifiers may be used per procedure, and should be written in column 24D on CMS-1500 claim form. CPT's Appendix A explains their use.

Categories II and III

Category II codes are optional and supplemental tracking codes. They track healthcare performance, programs, and counseling efforts. Example: Counseling to stop smoking.

Category III codes are temporary codes for emerging technologies, services, and procedures. Example: Implantation of an artificial heart. If possible, these codes should be used instead of the *unlisted codes* in the CPT.

> **Key Focus:** Category II and III codes are found after the final medicine codes in the CPT manual. *Unlisted codes* are rarely used, usually for new services or procedures that have not been assigned CPT codes.

Coding Terminology

Basic CPT coding terminology includes the following:

- Bundled codes—include more than one procedure; you should not unbundle procedures into component codes when a bundled procedure code is available; doing this is unethical and possibly fraudulent
- Concurrent care—similar care provided by more than one physician; usually involving several specialists

- Consultations—patient visits or appointments provided upon request of other healthcare providers; a service can only be considered a consultation with the "3Rs" present: *request* from another practitioner, *record* or documentation of findings and recommendations, and *reporting* to the referring practitioner
- Counseling—part of E/M services unless a complete history and physical exam do not occur; instead, *counseling* codes are used, such as for discussing concerns, test results, prognosis, risks, and education
- Critical care—for unstable, critically ill patients; constant bedside attention is required; the patient's condition must be critical in nature, but he or she does not need to be in a critical care or intensive care bed
- Downcoding—when the insurance carrier bases reimbursement on a code level lower than the one submitted by the provider; occurs due to unmatched coding systems, workers' compensation system differences, or when a payer requests medical records and finds they do not back up the level of code claimed
- Unbundling—breaking a bundled code into its component parts for higher reimbursement; not allowed
- Upcoding—coding at a higher level than the provided procedure or service, to receive a greater amount of reimbursement; also called *code creep*, *overbilling*, and *overcoding*; it is a fraudulent practice

Using the CPT Manual

When choosing E/M codes, you must know whether the patient is new or established, and where services occurred.

- Find the procedures and services provided—often these are on the superbill.

- Check patient chart to verify documentation of procedures, services in medical chart—if not written down, they did not occur.
- It may be easiest to go to the E/M section at the beginning of the CPT in order to choose the right code.
- For all other procedures, use the alphabetic listing of procedures in the back of the CPT manual.
- If a hyphen exists between two codes, there is a code range. Each code must be checked in numeric index.
- Code numbers with commas between them indicate more than one possible correct code location. Always check all possible codes.
- Check for any applicable modifiers. A modifier must be used if it is available for the situation.
- Enter the five-digit codes and modifiers in block 24D of the CMS-1500 form.
- Enter all other procedures provided on the date of service.
- Match all procedures with their appropriate diagnosis to verify medical necessity.

The HCPCS Coding Manual

The Healthcare Common Procedure Coding System, or HCPCS, was developed by the Centers for Medicare and Medicaid Services (CMS). Aside from Medicare and Medicaid, private insurers also accept certain HCPCS codes. Check with the insurer to see which HCPCS codes it accepts. There are two levels of the HCPCS:

- HCPCS Level I codes—more commonly known as CPT codes
- HCPCS Level II codes—national codes that cover supplies such as drugs, injections, durable medical equipment (DME), and sterile trays. If the CPT has a

generic description and the HCPCS has a more specific description, HCPCS Level II should be used.

- Level II codes also cover services and procedures not included in the CPT. It lists very specific codes for many different types of medical supplies and materials.
- Level II codes have five characters; they can be numbers, letters, or combinations of both. Examples include
  - E0781—ambulatory infusion pump, single or multiple channels
  - G0008—administration of influenza virus vaccine
  - Q0091—screening Papanicolaou (Pap) smear; obtaining, preparing, and conveyance of cervical or vaginal smear to laboratory
- There may also be two-character modifiers, either two letters or a letter and a number. These modifiers are different from the CPT modifiers. They are used with Level II *and* CPT codes, however.

Coding Compliance

Although licensed practitioners are ultimately responsible for coding accuracy and compliance with regulations, it is important for medical assistants to have knowledge of these procedures. Claims and the process used to generate claims must comply with federal and state laws, as well as with requirements of payers.

Coding Linkage
Insurers analyze coding linkage, which is the connection between diagnostic and procedural information. They evaluate medical necessity of all reported charges. Consequences of inaccurate coding and incorrect billing may include

- Delays in claims processing and receipt of payment

- Denied claims
- Exclusion from insurance programs
- Fines or other types of sanctions
- Loss of hospital privileges
- Loss of license to practice medicine
- Prison sentences
- Reduced payments

Codes are checked against medical documents.
These key points are checked during a code review
(coding audit):

- Appropriate codes are used for patient: age, condition, gender, new or established patient
- Coded services must be billable
- Diagnosis and procedure are clearly, correctly linked
- Diagnosis and procedure rules, set by payer, are followed
- Documentation in medical record supports reported services
- Reported services comply with all regulations

Evaluation and Management Services

Evaluation and management service codes under the CPT coding system are initially the most complex section to learn. They are also the most important. Evaluation and management codes are based on

- The patient's history—new patient or established patient; separate codes are used for each
- The degree of difficulty in medical decision making (the most complex part)
- The complexity of the examination

Evaluation and management codes link diagnoses and procedures with the amount of time a physician requires to correctly diagnose and treat a patient. There are four levels of decision making, as follows:

- Highly complex—patient is at high risk for complication or death if not treated
- Moderately complex—patient's condition has a moderate risk of complication or death if not treated
- Less complex—low risk of complication or death if not treated
- Straightforward—minimal risk of complication or death if not treated

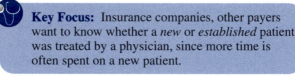

Key Focus: Insurance companies, other payers want to know whether a *new* or *established* patient was treated by a physician, since more time is often spent on a new patient.

Different E/M codes apply to services performed in these specific locations:

- The offices of physicians
- Emergency rooms in hospitals
- Inpatient hospital rooms
- Facilities that offer extended care
- Nursing homes
- Patients' homes

Table 9-4 explains a breakdown of evaluation and management codes.

Key Focus: DSM-IV codes are part of the *Diagnostic and Statistical Manual of Mental Disorders, 4th Edition, Text Revision*, or *DSM-IV-TR*. Published by the American Psychiatric Association, it includes all currently recognized mental health disorders, and corresponds with ICD-10 codes.

Diagnostic

Table 9-4 *E/M Code Breakdown*

Code Range	Type of Services
99201–99205 (new patient) 99211–99215 (established patient)	Office/Other Outpatient Services
99217–99226	Hospital Observation Services
99221–99239	Hospital Inpatient Services
99241–99245 (outpatient) 99251–99255 (inpatient)	Consultations
99281–99288	Emergency Department Services
99291–99292	Critical Care Services
99304–99318	Nursing Facility Services
99324–99328 (new patient) 99334–99337 (established patient)	Domiciliary, Rest Home (Boarding Home), or Custodial Care Services
99339–99340	Domiciliary, Assisted Living Facility, or Home Care Plan Oversight Services
99341–99345 (new patient) 99347–99350 (established patient)	Home Services

(*continued*)

Table 9-4 (*Continued*)

Code Range	Type of Services
99354–99360	Prolonged Services
99363–99368	Case Management Services
99375–99380	Care Plan Oversight Services
99381–99387 (new patient) 99391–99397 (established patient) 99420–99429 (other)	Preventative Medicine Services (Includes Counseling Services)
99441–99449	Non-Face-to-Face Physician Services
99450–99456	Special Evaluation and Management Services
99460–99465	Newborn Care Services
99466–99486	Inpatient Neonatal Intensive Care Services and Pediatric and Neonatal Critical Care Services
99487–99490	Care Management Services
99495–99496	Transitional Care Management Services
99497–99498	Advance Care Planning
99499	Other Evaluation and Management Services

SECTION III
Clinical Medical Assisting

Clinical Medical
Assisting

CHAPTER 10
Infection Control and Principles of Asepsis

Medical assistants play an essential role in controlling and preventing the spread of infection. Infection control involves the following:

- Chain of infection, also known as the *cycle of infection*
- The Occupational Safety and Health Administration (OSHA) Bloodborne Pathogens standard
- Standard precautions
- Transmission-based precautions
- OSHA-required education and training for healthcare workers

RISK FACTORS FOR HEALTHCARE-ASSOCIATED INFECTIONS

Patients can acquire infections as a result of many different types of healthcare facilities. Common risk factors for health-associated infections include

- Communicable disease transmission between patients and healthcare workers (e.g., influenza)
- Contamination from healthcare environment
- Immunocompromised patients
- Improper use of antibiotics
- Surgical procedures
- Use of indwelling devices like catheters (fixed inside the body for a period of time)

THE CHAIN OF INFECTION

Knowledge of the chain of infection facilitates control or prevention of disease by breaking the links in the chain:

- Reservoir host (agents)
  - Biological agents
  - Chemical agents
  - Physical agents
- Means of exit
- Means of transmission
  - After taking care of an infected patient
  - Between contacts with high-risk patients
  - Immediately after gloves are removed
  - Before and after performing sterile procedures
  - After contact with blood or body substances, waste, or contaminated equipment
- Means of entrance
- Susceptible host

Key Focus: To break the chain of infection and its spread, you must apply the principles of asepsis.

PRINCIPLES OF ASEPSIS

The most effective way to eliminate the transmission of disease from one host to another is through asepsis, which means "being completely sterile" (free from microorganisms).

PERSONAL PROTECTIVE EQUIPMENT

Personal protective equipment (PPE) is protective gear worn to guard against physical hazards. It includes

- Face shields
- Gloves

- Gowns
- Masks
- Protective eyewear

MEDICAL ASEPSIS

Medical asepsis is also called *clean technique*, which includes cleaning, disinfection, hand hygiene, and sanitizing.

Cleansing Agents

The following are some examples of agents used for cleansing the hands:

- Alcohol or alcohol-based products
- Antimicrobial foams
- Chlorhexidine gluconate
- Hexachlorophene
- Iodine/iodophor agents
- Plain soap

Hand Hygiene

- Before and after touching wounds
- Before and after assisting with any surgery
- Before and after taking care of any patient, including particularly susceptible patients, such as newborns or severely immunocompromised patients
- Between patient contacts

PROCEDURE 10-1 *Hand Hygiene*

1. Remove watches, rings, and bracelets.
2. Inspect the hands for any breaks in the skin.
3. Turn on the faucets and check the water temperature.

4. Keep the hands upright.
5. Allow the water to run over the hands.
6. Apply approved hand-cleaning substances.
7. Apply friction on all surfaces of the hands and fingers.
8. Wash all surfaces of the hands and under the nails for 2 minutes.
9. Rinse thoroughly with a flowing stream of water.
10. The fingertips should be pointing down.
11. Most healthcare professionals suggest that the hands should be thoroughly washed for between 30 seconds and 1 minute.

Key Focus: The faucets, if not foot or knee operated, should be turned off using a paper towel.

SURGICAL ASEPSIS

It refers to maintaining a sterile environment or destruction of all organisms before they enter the body. Three methods used for preventing disease spread in medical workplaces: sanitization, disinfection, sterilization.

Sanitization

Sanitization is a way of inhibiting or inactivating pathogens by washing and scrubbing instruments, equipment by

1. Using a brush with hot water and a soapless cleaner
2. Using ultrasound cleaning methods

Disinfection

Disinfection is a process that eliminates many or all pathogenic microorganisms, but is not effective against spores.

Factors That Affect Disinfection

- Previous cleaning of the object
- Type and level of microbial contamination
- Concentration, exposure time to germicides
- Temperature, pH of the disinfection process
- Physical configuration of objects, such as hinges, lumens, and crevices

Chemical Disinfectant Agents

- Soap
- Alcohols (70% isopropyl)
- Phenol
- Formaldehyde
- Chlorine
- Hydrogen peroxide
- Peracetic acid
- Peracetic acid with hydrogen peroxide

Key Focus: Topical antimicrobial and antiseptic products are recommended for use in surgical settings.

PROCEDURE 10-2 *Surgical Scrubbing*

Remove debris from the nails, hands, and forearms.

1. Remove all jewelry from the fingers, hands, and forearms.
2. Keep fingernails short, clean, and healthy.
3. Do not wear artificial nails.
4. Wash hands and forearms vigorously.
5. Scrub hands and forearms, moving up to and including the elbows; spend 5 minutes on each arm.

6. Apply an antimicrobial agent.
7. Vigorously scrub the four sides of the fingers, hands, and arms.
8. Hold the hands higher than the elbows.
9. Raise hands and place them under running water to rinse off soap.
10. If required by the surgical procedure, scrub each hand for 3 minutes with a brush.
11. After scrubbing, keep the hands up and away from the body.
12. Turn off faucet with a fresh towel if a foot lever is not available.
13. Dry the hands and arms with a sterile towel.
14. Glove immediately; keep hands above the waist, folded together until the procedure begins.

Key Focus: The optimum duration of scrubbing is not known. Recommendations, however, are for a 2- to 5-minute surgical scrub using an appropriate antiseptic.

Sterilization

Sterilization destroys all microorganisms, including spores. Sterilization can be accomplished by heat (steam or dry), chemical agents, high-velocity electron bombardment, or ultraviolet light radiation. Physical sterilization uses steam sterilization, dry sterilization, or prevacuum sterilization.

Steam Sterilization (Autoclaves)

Methods used for sterilization include the autoclave and chemical (cold) sterilization. The most common steam-sterilizing temperatures are 250°F (121°C) and 270°F (132°C). Sterilization times vary, based on type of item, wrapped items, unwrapped items, and type of sterilizer. Table 10-1 describes autoclave sterilization time requirements.

Table 10-1 *Sterilization Times*

Items to Be Sterilized	Time Required (minutes)
Glassware	15
Metal instruments—open tray or individualized wrapping with hinges open	
Needles	
Syringes	
Instruments—partial metal in double-thickness wrapper or covered tray	20
Rubber products—catheters, gloves, tubing—wrapped or unwrapped	
Solutions in a flask (50–100 mL)	
Dressings—small packs in muslin or paper	30
Gauze—loosely packed	
Instrument and treatment trays—wrapped in muslin or paper	
Needles—individually packaged in glass tubes or paper	
Solutions in a flask (500–1,000 mL)	
Sutures—wrapper in muslin or paper	
Syringes—unassembled, wrapped individually in gauze	
Syringes—unassembled, wrapped individually in glass tubes	
Petroleum jelly—in dry heat	60

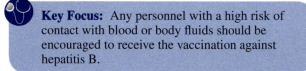

Key Focus: After autoclaving, instrument packages are considered sterile for 21 days (in plastic bags) to 30 days (in muslin), with a shelf life of approximately 1 month.

BLOODBORNE PATHOGENS AND SAFETY ISSUES

Three well-known bloodborne diseases include

1. Acquired immunodeficiency syndrome (AIDS)
2. Hepatitis B (HBV)
3. Hepatitis C (HCV)

The OSHA Bloodborne Pathogen Rule is based on the Centers for Disease Control and Prevention's concept of "standard precautions," to prevent bloodborne pathogen transmission in the workplace.

Body fluids that apply to standard precautions include

- Amniotic fluid
- Blood products
- Semen and vaginal secretions
- Cerebrospinal fluid
- Pericardial fluid
- Peritoneal fluid
- Pleural fluid
- Spinal fluid
- Synovial fluid

Key Focus: Any personnel with a high risk of contact with blood or body fluids should be encouraged to receive the vaccination against hepatitis B.

Standard precautions should also be followed when handling

- Feces
- Nasal secretions
- Saliva
- Sputum
- Sweat
- Breast milk
- Tears
- Urine
- Vomitus

General Safety Practice Guidelines

- Used injection needles should not be recapped except by using a recapping safety device.
- Needles should not be removed from a disposable syringe after use. Dispose them as a unit.
- Needles and sutures should be manipulated with forceps rather than with gloved fingers.
- Sharps should not be manipulated by hand.
- All blades and needles must be placed in a puncture-resistant sharps disposal container.

Written Exposure Plan

OSHA requires medical facilities to have a written exposure control plan (ECP). Employees at risk of bloodborne exposure must have access to the plan. It must be reviewed with new employees upon employment and with all employees every year. Written copies must be given to employees requesting them. An ECP must include

- Determination of employee exposure
- Implementation of exposure control methods:
  - Universal precautions

- Engineering and work practice controls
- Housekeeping
- Personal protective equipment
- Hepatitis B vaccination
- Postexposure evaluation, follow-up
- Hazard communication for employees; hazard training
- Recordkeeping
- Procedures about evaluating exposure incidents and their circumstances

Exposure Incidents

Exposure incidents are those in which an employee, even when precautions were taken, believes that he or she has come into contact with a potentially infectious substance, such as through a needlestick.

- Puncture exposures are the most common type.
- Rules apply to HIV, HBV, and other serious infections.
- The physician or employer must be notified immediately.
- Quick, proper treatment is essential to prevent disease, or spreading of a disease to others.
- Reporting also reduces chances for future incidents.
- Free medical evaluations must be offered by employers.
- Blood samples are taken and treatments are provided.
- Employees can refuse evaluation and treatment, but this must be documented by the employer.
- If HBV is involved, the employee should be tested and receive vaccination if necessary.

Needlestick Safety and Prevention Act

This Act revised OSHA's Bloodborne Pathogens standard.

- Protective safety devices must be evaluated annually.
- Detailed *sharps injury logs* must be maintained.

- Employees should help identify, evaluate, and implement engineering and work practice controls.
- Engineering controls eliminate use of needles where safe, effective alternatives are available.
- Engineered safety devices must be evaluated regularly.
- Prevention programs help to
  - Identify hazard trends
  - Ensure proper training
  - Adapt practices to make use of sharps safer
  - Heighten safety awareness
  - Establish strict procedures for reporting needlesticks
  - Evaluate prevention procedures while providing feedback to employees

CHAPTER 11
Minor Surgery

THE ROLE OF MEDICAL ASSISTANTS IN MINOR SURGERY

- Assisting the physician
- Following the guidelines for surgical asepsis
- Setting up the operating room
- Setting up surgical instruments and supplies
- Preparing the sterile field
- Preparing the patient for surgery
- Draping the incision site
- Measuring vital signs
- Passing instruments
- Operating suction machines
- Preparing specimens for the laboratory
- Cutting sutures
- Dressing the patient's wound
- Restocking operating room supplies

CLASSIFICATIONS OF SURGICAL INSTRUMENTS

Various instruments are used for the many different procedures in minor surgeries. These instruments may be designed for

- Cutting
- Dissecting

- Grasping
- Clamping
- Probing
- Dilating
- Retracting
- Suturing

Cutting Instruments

- Scalpels or knives
  - A scalpel blade is inserted into the scalpel handle
  - Figure 11-1 (see student resources website) shows a variety of scalpels and blades
- Scissors
  - Operating or suture scissors
  - Dissecting or straight (Mayo) scissors
  - Bandage scissors

Grasping Instruments

Forceps are used to grasp tissue or objects. Types of forceps are summarized in Table 11-1.

Surgical Trays

Surgical trays generally contain various instruments and materials, including

- Scissors
- Several pairs of forceps
- Hemostats
- Needle holders
- Suture material
- Sterile gauze

Table 11-1 *Types of Forceps and Their Indications*

Types	Uses
Hemostat forceps	Applied to a blood vessel to stop bleeding
Needle holder forceps	Grasping needles during suturing
Thumb forceps	Holding tissue
Tissue forceps	Grasping tissue
Splinter forceps	Grasping foreign bodies
Sponge forceps	Holding sponges during surgery
Towel forceps	Holding the edges of sterile drapes together

Probing and Dilating Instruments

Some instruments are used to enter body cavities for probing or dilating. They include

- Laryngoscopes (see Figure 11-2a and b on student resources website)—used for visual examination of the voice box area
- Speculums (see Figure 11-3)—used for enlarging the opening of any canal or cavity of the body for inspection of its interior
- Probes (see Figure 11-4 on student resources website)—used for detection of a substance or for exploration of an area
- Trocars (see Figure 11-5 on student resources website)—used for withdrawing fluid from a cavity
- Punches—used to directly pierce an organ or through the skin

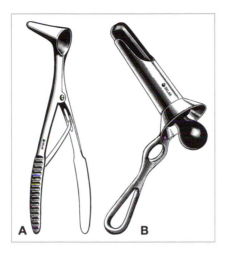

Figure 11–3 *Speculums: (A) Vienna nasal;*
(B) Ives-Fanster rectal.

- Retractors—used for drawing aside edges of a wound, or holding back structures near operative field

Suturing Instruments

Suturing instruments are used to tie tissues and other body components together and may be made of absorbable or nonabsorbable materials. Suture materials include the following:

- Silk
- Nylon
- Polyester
- Cotton
- Steel

Suture Sizes

They are determined by a gauge or diameter, starting in terms of zeros (0s) and decreasing in size with number of zeros added. "0" is the thickest and "6-0" (000000) is the smallest. Table 11-2 summarizes various types, sizes, and indications of sutures.

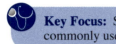

Key Focus: Sizes 2-0 through 6-0 are most commonly used.

Table 11-2 *Various Types of Suture Materials, Sizes, and Indications*

Types of Material	Sizes	Indications
Chromic gut	3-0 to 0	Blood vessels
Cotton	3-0	
Silk	3-0 to 0	
Chromic gut	2-0 to 0	Facial
Cotton	2-0 to 0	
Silk	2-0 to 0	
Nylon	6-0 to 2-0	Skin
Polyethylene	5-0 to 3-0	
Stainless steel	5-0 to 2-0	
Chromic gut	3-0 to 0	Muscle
Plain gut	3-0 to 0	
Silk	3-0 to 0	

SURGICAL SETUP

A surgical setup for a typical minor surgical procedure includes

- Local anesthetic materials
- Alcohol sponges to clean vial tops
- Syringes with needles
- Sterile gloves
- Gauze sponges
- Scalpel blades, handles (numbers 3, 10, 11, 15)
- Curved iris scissors
- Towel forceps
- Tissue forceps
- Straight and curved Kelly forceps
- Straight and curved mosquito forceps
- Sterile drape towels
- Sterile specimen containers with preservative solution
- Needle holders with mounted needles
- Suture materials

Handling Instruments

Properly caring for each surgical instrument is essential. After the surgical procedure, you must

- Unlock instruments before immersion.
- Never allow blood to dry on an instrument because it is difficult to remove.
- Place instruments in a basin of disinfectant solution.
- Place heavier instruments at the bottom of the basin, with more delicate instruments on top.
- Thoroughly scrub, rinse instruments with a neutral pH detergent solution and a soft brush.
- Rinse instruments with distilled water.
- Dry instruments with a lint-free cloth, or allow them to air dry.
- Package instruments for sterilization.

Minor Surgery

SUTURE REMOVAL

Sutures remain in place from 2 to 10 days; they must be removed if nonabsorbable. Suture removal times differ:

- Head and neck sutures remain for 3–5 days.
- Facial sutures can be removed after only 24–48 hours to prevent scarring.
- Abdominal sutures remain for 5–7 days.
- Sutures on knee joints and large bones may remain for 7–10 days.

SPECIAL SURGICAL PROCEDURES

Many minor surgical procedures are performed in the medical office and may require anesthetics, either injected locally at site of the procedure or sprayed onto the skin as preinjection anesthesia. Surgeries performed in the office:

- Biopsy—removal of a small piece of tissue, then examining it under a microscope to confirm a diagnosis
- Irrigation—cleaning of a puncture wound
- Colposcopy—visual examination of the vagina and cervix with a colposcope
- Cryosurgery—a noninvasive treatment that uses subfreezing temperatures to freeze and destroy tissue
- Laser surgery—use of surgical lasers to conduct procedures in lieu of standard equipment (such as scalpels)
- Curettage—the process of scraping material from the wall of a cavity for the purpose of removing abnormal tissue
- Endoscopy—a procedure using a flexible tube that may contain a tiny camera, blade, cauterizing (burning) device
- Removal of foreign bodies
- Suture removal

- Vasectomy—a surgical cutting and tying of the vas deferens to prevent the passage of sperm
- Removal of small tumors

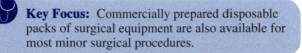

Key Focus: Commercially prepared disposable packs of surgical equipment are also available for most minor surgical procedures.

Visit www.pearsonhighered.com/healthprofessionsresources to access figures and tables available on the student resources website. Click on view all resources and select Medical Assisting from the choice of disciplines. Find this book and you can see all respective tables and figures.

Minor Surgery

CHAPTER 12

Vital Signs and Preparing the Patient

Vital signs include temperature (T), pulse (P), respiration (R), and blood pressure (BP).

> **Key Focus:** When taking vital signs, the medical assistant should weigh the patient on a medical office scale and measure height using the height bar attached to scale.

FACTORS AFFECTING VITAL SIGNS

- Age
- Gender
- Race and heredity
- Medications
- Environment
- Pain
- Lifestyle
- Biological rhythms
  - Blood pressure is lowest in the morning and peaks in the late afternoon and evening
  - Temperature is highest in the evening and lowest in the early morning

> **Key Focus:** African-Americans are more prone to high BP, resulting from increased salt sensitivity or increased blood cholesterol levels.

NORMAL VITAL SIGNS IN PEDIATRIC PATIENTS

A summary of normal vital signs in pediatric patients is shown in Table 12-1.

Key Focus: Medical assistants should always consider the culture, religion, age, and gender of patients when taking their vital signs.

TEMPERATURE

Fever is considered to be above-normal body temperature. Body temperature is measured with a thermometer.

Key Focus: Mercury thermometers are no longer used in healthcare due to potential dangers of mercury and frequency of breakage. Mercury is toxic to humans and animals.

Table 12-1 *Normal Vital Signs for Pediatric Patients*

Age	Normal Pulse Range	Normal Pulse Average	BP (Average)	Respiration (Average)
Newborn	110–180	140	90/55	30–50
1 year	80–150	120	90/60	20–40
2 years	83–130	110	95/60	20–30
4 years	80–120	100	99/65	20–25
6 years	75–115	100	100/56	20–25
8 years	70–110	90	105/56	15–20
10 years	70–110	90	110/58	15–20

Vital Signs

Table 12-2 *Comparisons of Body Temperatures Between Fahrenheit and Celsius*

Type	Fahrenheit	Celsius
Oral	98.6	37.0
Tympanic	99.6	37.6
Axillary	97.6	36.6
Rectal	99.6	38.6

Measuring Temperature

- Normal body temperature range: 97°F to 99°F (36°C to 37.2°C). Average temperature is 98.6°F (or 37°C). Table 12-2 compares average temperatures of body areas.
- Celsius or centigrade (C): 0°C is freezing point of water (sea level) and 100°C is boiling point of water (sea level).
- Fahrenheit (F): Boiling point of water is 212°F (sea level) and 32°F is freezing point of water (sea level).
- Conversion formulas: Two formulas are used to compare the Celsius and Fahrenheit temperatures:
  - To convert Celsius to Fahrenheit: $F = (C \times 9/5) + 32$
  - To convert Fahrenheit to Celsius: $C = (F - 32) \times 5/9$

Appendix I compares Celsius (centigrade) and Fahrenheit temperatures.

Thermometers and Temperatures

- Electronic or digital thermometers: considered accurate, easy to read, sanitary, fast, and easy to clean.
  - Equipped with two probes:
    - Blue (for oral or axillary)
    - Red (for rectal)

- Measure temperature within 10–60 seconds
- Disposable probe covers are placed over the thermometer for each use

Key Focus: The electronic thermometer unit should always be returned to the charging stand after each use to maintain the battery.

- Tympanic thermometers: advised for patients over 3 months of age and used for quick, safe, and accurate measurement of body temperature, via the ear canal. Advantages include
  - Temperature obtained in less than 2 seconds
  - Popular with patients due to comfort of use

Key Focus: Do not use ear thermometers in infected or draining ears, or if adjacent lesions or incisions exist.

- Axillary temperature: often used for children who are unconscious or who have a structural abnormality.
  - Accurate as long as technique is performed correctly; oral or rectal thermometers are more accurate.
  - Take more time to get the result (though usually less than 1 minute, if using a digital thermometer).
  - Commonly used for newborns, infants, children, and adults with jaw impairments or surgery.

Key Focus: The temperature of an unconscious client is never taken by mouth. The rectal, axillary, or tympanic methods are preferred.

- Rectal temperature: when using a digital thermometer, for a rectal temperature, the reading is usually complete in less than 1 minute. They are used
  - For infants
  - When tympanic thermometers are not available
  - When the patient has breathing difficulties
  - For unconscious patients

Key Focus: Rectal temperatures are usually 1° more than oral temperatures and 2° more than axillary temperatures.

- Chemical thermometers: examples such as Traxlt chemical strip tape or liquid crystal thermometers are to be used for only one patient. They are placed either on the forehead or under the tongue (see Figure 12-1). For this method, you should consider the following:
  - Readings are obtained by heat-sensitive bars or patches
  - Changes color to indicate body temperature

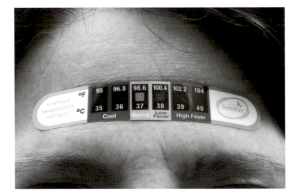

Figure 12-1 *Chemical thermometer on the forehead.*

- Commonly used for young children, and also at home
- Least accurate type as compared to digital or tympanic thermometers
- Temperature is usually measured within 15 seconds

Key Focus: It is important to check the expiration dates and storage restrictions of chemical thermometers to ensure their accuracy.

PULSE

Pulse is the expansion of an artery caused by flow of blood when the heart beats. The number of beats in a minute is called the pulse rate. See Table 12-3 for normal pulse rates. Many factors affect pulse rate:

- Gender
- Body size
- Physical exercise
- Health status
- Drugs
- Age

Table 12-3 *Normal Pulse Rate Averages*

Age Group	Range (beats/minute)
Newborn to 1 year	120–160
2–6 years	80–120
6–10 years	80–100
11–16 years	70–90
Adult	60–80
Older adult	50–65

Vital Signs

> **Key Focus:** Infants and children have a faster pulse than adults, and women have a faster pulse than men.

Pulse Sites

- Radial—the inner part of the forearm on the thumb side of the wrist; most commonly used site
- Apical—at the apex of the heart, to the left of the sternum; used frequently for infants and elderly persons
- Carotid—used when other sites are inaccessible
- Brachial—inner part of the elbow
- Temporal—at the side of the head, just above the ear
- Femoral—in the groin, where the femoral artery passes to the leg
- Popliteal—behind the knee
- Dorsalis pedis—on top of the foot, slightly lateral to the midline for pulse sites

See Figure 12-2 for pulse sites.

> **Key Focus:** Femoral, popliteal, and pedal pulses can be hard to find. A Doppler ultrasound stethoscope helps by magnifying these pulsations, and is battery-operated.

Characteristics of Pulse

The following are important characteristics of pulse:

- Rate: rate of the pulse as observed in an artery (normally, it is the same as the heart rate)
- Rhythm: the regular or irregular sequence of pulses that make up the pulse rate
- Volume: the capacity or strength of the pulses

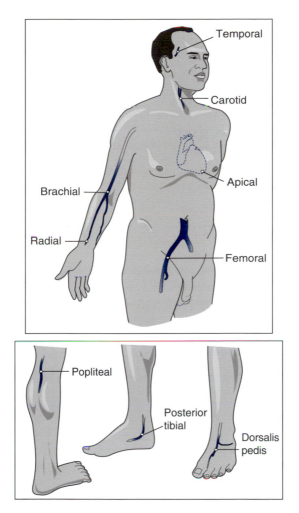

Figure 12-2 *Pulse sites.*

- Compliance of arteries (elasticity): quality of being able to return to original shape after being compressed, bent, or otherwise distorted

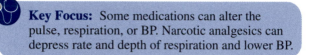

Key Focus: Some medications can alter the pulse, respiration, or BP. Narcotic analgesics can depress rate and depth of respiration and lower BP.

RESPIRATION RATE

A *respiration* consists of one inhalation and one exhalation. The normal respiratory rates are summarized in Table 12-4.

The important characteristics of respirations include

- Rate: number of respirations per minute
- Rhythm: the breathing pattern
- Depth: amount of air being inhaled and exhaled
- Chest wall movements: the observation of the movement of the chest wall

Key Focus: Respirations should be counted for a full minute rather than for 15 or 30 seconds.

Table 12-4 *Normal Respiratory Rates in Different Ages*

Age	Range (breaths/minute)
Newborns	30–50
Infants	20–40
Children (1–9 years)	20–30
Children (11–18 years)	18–24
Adults	14–20

Breath Sounds

Normal respirations have no noticeable sound. Breath sounds occur in some disease conditions. Table 12-5 lists common breath sounds.

Table 12-5 *Common Breath Sounds*

Terms	Sounds	Examples
Stridor	A shrill, harsh sound heard more clearly during inspiration	Croup, laryngeal obstruction
Stertorous	Noisy breathing sounds	Snoring
Crackles (rales)	Crackling sounds resembling crushing tissue paper	Pneumonia
Rhonchi	Also called gurgles; rattling, whistling sounds made in the throat	Tracheostomy requires suctioning
Wheezes	High-pitched, whistling sounds made when airway becomes obstructed	Asthma or COPD
Bubbling	Breathing sounds like gurgling sounds; as if air is passing through moist secretions in respiratory tract	Tracheostomy

Table 12-6 *Normal Blood Pressure at Various Ages*

Age	Systolic/Diastolic (mmHg)
Newborn	75/55
Child (6–9 years of age)	90/55
Child (10–15 years of age)	100/65
Adolescent (16–17 years of age)	118/76
Adult (18 years of age and up)	120/80
Prehypertension	120–139/80–89
Hypertension	Above 140/90

BLOOD PRESSURE

Blood pressure (BP) is the force that blood exerts against the walls of the arteries. Table 12-6 lists the normal BP at various ages.

Factors Affecting Blood Pressure

The following physiological factors can change BP:

- Blood volume
- Peripheral resistance of the vessels
- Vessel elasticity
- Blood viscosity
- Condition of the heart muscle

Key Focus: Avoid measuring BP in an arm with extensive axillary node dissection, such as with radical mastectomy.

Table 12-7 *Blood Pressure Cuff Sizes*

Age	Size
Newborn	5–7.5 cm wide
Infant	7.5–13 cm wide
Child	13–20 cm wide (The cuff size for a child should cover 2/3 of the upper arm.)
Average adult	24–32 cm wide (Adult cuffs should have a width that covers 1/3 to 1/2 of the circumference of the arm; the length of the bladder should cover about 80% of the arm—which is about twice the size of the width.)
Large adult	32–42 cm wide

Measuring Blood Pressure

The point at which the heartbeat is first heard is the systolic pressure; the point at which the sound disappears is the diastolic pressure. Table 12-7 lists guidelines for sphygmomanometer selection.

Key Focus: When a client moves from recumbent to standing position, systolic pressure can fall 10–15 mmHg and diastolic pressure may rise by 5 mmHg.

Korotkoff Sounds
Korotkoff sounds are the actual sounds heard as the arterial wall distends during the compression of the BP

Table 12-8 *Korotkoff Phases of Blood Pressure Sounds*

Phase	Sound
I	Faint tapping heard when cuff deflates (systolic BP)
II	Soft swishing sounds
III	Rhythmic, sharp, crisp tapping
IV	Soft tapping sounds that become muffled
V	Last sound disappears (diastolic BP)

cuff. Korotkoff sounds consist of five distinct phases (see Table 12-8).

Key Focus: The American Heart Association recommends routine use of the *bell* of the stethoscope for BP (Korotkoff sounds) auscultation.

THE PATIENT EXAM AND POSITIONING

Different physical examinations require the patient to be placed into specific positions.

Equipment Required for Physical Examinations

The following equipment is found in the examining room:

- Stethoscope
- Sphygmomanometer
- Otoscope
- Ophthalmoscope
- Nasal speculum
- Laryngeal mirror

- Reflex hammer with pinwheel
- Tuning fork
- Tape measure
- Tongue depressor
- Gloves
- Vaginal speculum or histobrush
- Flashlight or penlight
- Lubricant
- Cotton applicators
- Emesis basin
- Gauze sponges
- Tonometer
- Alcohol wipes
- Snellen chart
- Ishihara color plates
- Balance scale
- Disposable pads
- Gowns for patients
- Drapes

Key Focus: Gauze squares, cotton balls, cotton-tipped applicators, glass slides, and laboratory request forms should all be readily available for use during an examination.

Methods of Examination

The six commonly used methods of physical examination include

- Inspection: visual examination of the patient's body and overall appearance
- Auscultation: listening to body sounds using a stethoscope (the heart, lungs, and abdominal organs)
- Palpation: using the hands to feel the skin and accessible underlying organs

- Percussion: tapping or striking the body lightly to gain information about the position and size of the underlying body parts (or to feel vibrations, such as whether the lungs contain air or fluid)
- Manipulation: for example, accessing the range of motion of a joint
- Mensuration: the process of measuring the body or specific body parts (such as weight and height)

Draping the Patient

Always offer a gown or drape to each patient. Older adults may need assistance with undressing and draping.

> **Key Focus:** Never turn your back on a seriously ill or disoriented patient. The same is true for young children. Ensure patient safety at all times.

Positioning the Patient

A variety of patient positions are used to assist the physician in performing physical examinations. Table 12-9 summarizes the various types of positioning and their indications. Figure 12-3 shows the various positions that may be used during the physical examination.

Positioning Procedures for Assisting the Physician

- Identify the patient
- Explain the rationale for the procedure
- Select the appropriate position for specific physical examination
- Choose the appropriate gown
- Cover the patient with a drape
- Hand instruments and equipment to the physician as needed

Table 12-9 *Positions and Indications*

Positions	Indications (Uses)
Dorsal recumbent	Digital exams of the vagina and rectum
Fowler's	Examination of the head, neck, and upper body
Knee-chest	Proctologic exams, sigmoidoscopy procedure, and rectal or vaginal exams
Lithotomy	Vaginal examinations (when a vaginal speculum must be used) and Pap smears
Proctologic jackknife	Sigmoidoscopy
Prone	Used for back exams and certain types of surgery
Semi-Fowler's	Used for postsurgical exams and for breathing difficulties
Sims' (lateral)	Rectal exams, taking rectal temperature, enemas, and pelvic exams
Sitting	Examination of the patient's head, neck, chest, heart, back, and arms
Supine (horizontal recumbent)	Examination of the head, chest, stomach, and also used for x-rays
Trendelenburg	Abdominal surgeries

Vital Signs

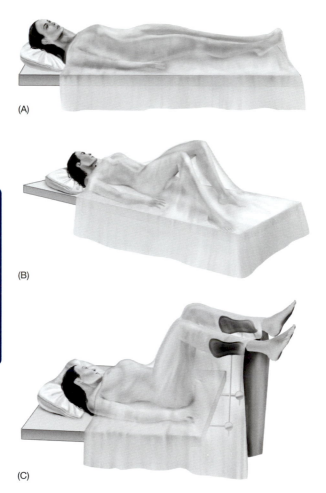

Figure 12-3 *(A) Supine or horizontal recumbent, (B) dorsal recumbent, (C) lithotomy, (Continued)*

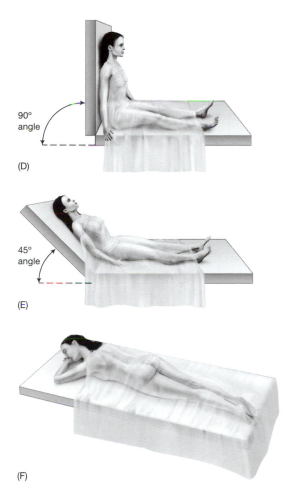

(D)

(E)

(F)

Figure 12-3 *(D) Fowler's, (E) semi-Fowler's, (F) prone, (Continued)*

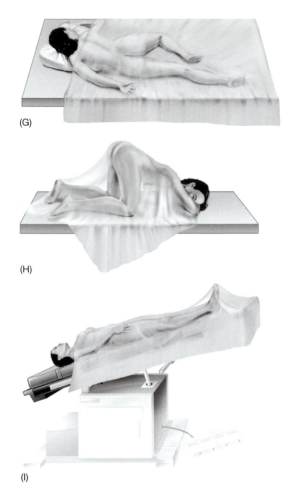

(G)

(H)

(I)

Figure 12-3 *(G) Sims' or lateral, (H) knee-chest, (I) Trendelenburg, (Continued)*

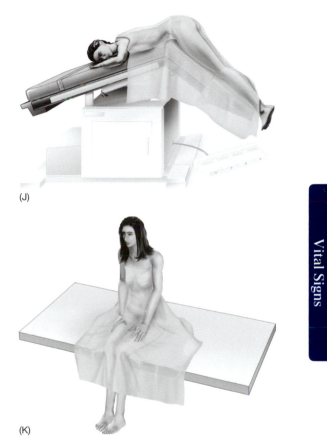

(J)

(K)

Vital Signs

Figure 12-3 *(J) proctologic (jack-knife), and (K) sitting.*
(*Continued*)

- Document and label specimens
- Act as a witness to the examination
- Carry out treatment plans by
  - Providing patient education
  - Applying dressings
  - Administering medications
- Schedule diagnostic tests (as ordered by the physician)

Sequence of Examination Procedures

Typically, examination procedures follow this sequence:

- Taking the medical history of the patient
- Identifying the chief complaint and history of the current illness
- Reviewing of systems (head-to-toe exam):
  - Skin, hair, and nails
  - Head, neck, eyes, ears, nose, mouth, and throat
  - Arms, heart, chest, and lungs
  - Abdomen, genitalia, rectum, legs, and feet
  - Neurological system

Chapter 13
Electrocardiography

The physician may order a test to monitor the heart of a patient when heart sounds are unusual, the rhythm is irregular, the patient has any heart-related complaints, or the patient has a condition related to the heart. Most often, it is the medical assistant who will perform these tests.

THE ELECTROCARDIOGRAM (ECG, EKG)

ECGs may be used to assist in diagnosing the following disorders or conditions:

- Ischemia of the heart muscle (heart attack)
- Delays in impulse conduction
- Hypertrophy of the cardiac chambers
- Arrhythmias (to identify irregularities in heart rhythms)

Equipment

For performing an ECG, the following equipment is required:

- Electrocardiograph paper
- Electrodes or sensors (which receive electrical impulses)
- Lead wires (which attach to electrodes)
- ECG machine

See Figure 13-1 for a depiction of the heart and an ECG tracing, with the various waves signified.

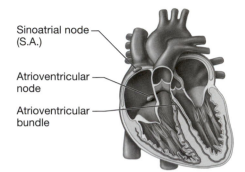

Sinoatrial node
(S.A.)

Atrioventricular
node

Atrioventricular
bundle

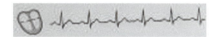

S.A. Node

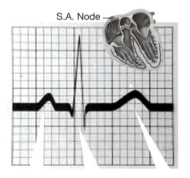

P wave	**QRS complex**	**T wave**
corresponds to contraction of the atria	correlates to ventricles contracting	represents preparation for next series of complexes

Figure 13-1 *The heart and electrocardiogram tracing.*

Electrocardiography

Electrodes and Leads

Electrodes (sensors) identify the electrical impulses on the body surface through wires attached to the ECG machine. There are a series of lead wires that come from the ECG machine, which are connected to the electrodes or sensors. These lead wires provide the circuit from the patient to the machine.

Sensor Position

A sensor is a device designed to respond to electrical impulses of the heart. The standard ECG consists of 12 leads and 10 sensors. The sensors are placed on the patient's upper arms or both forearms, the inner aspects of both lower legs, and on the chest, as follows:

- Right arm (RA)
- Left arm (LA)
- Left leg (LL)
- Right leg (RL)
- V leads (C leads) or chest (or precordial) leads

Key Focus: The RL sensor serves as an electrical reference point and is not actually used in the recording. It is also called the ground sensor.

ECG Leads

The standard ECG records depolarization and repolarization along designated paths called *leads*. A medical assistant should be familiar with the following terms:

- Lead: an electrical picture of the heart's surface
- Electrodes: the two points between which the electrical activity occurs

- Bipolar leads: the electrodes have opposite polarity (one is positive, another is negative)
- Unipolar leads: made up of one positive electrode and another that is used as a reference point

Standard Leads

There are 12 individual leads in the standard ECG, which include

- Six limb leads
  - Three leads (standard leads)
  - Three unipolar leads (augmented leads)
- Six precordial leads (unipolar) or chest leads

Limb Leads

The limb leads include I, II, III (standard leads), and aVR, aVL, and aVF (augmented leads). Table 13-1 shows the limb leads and the surface viewed.

The limb leads represent a triangle, called Einthoven's triangle (see Figure 13-2).

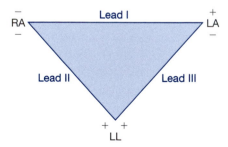

Figure 13-2 *Einthoven's triangle.*

Table 13-1 *Limb Leads and Surfaces Viewed*

Lead	Surface Viewed
I	Left heart wall
II	Inferior, apical
III	Right inferior wall

Augmented Leads

The augmented leads are a combination of the two limb leads angled 30° from each other. They include

- aVR
- aVL
- aVF

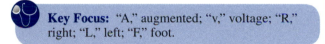 **Key Focus:** "A," augmented; "v," voltage; "R," right; "L," left; "F," foot.

Precordial (Chest) Leads

The six precordial leads are placed directly over the heart itself. These leads are known as V_1, V_2, V_3, V_4, V_5, and V_6. Figure 13-3 shows the precordial chest lead placements.

Table 13-2 summarizes the locations of the precordial electrodes.

Marking Code

There are many codes used to determine each lead recorded on an ECG reading. These codes are required for I.D. and mounting purposes. Table 13-3 shows sensor lead placement and a common coding system.

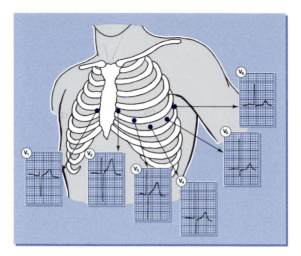

Figure 13-3 *Precordial chest lead placements.*

Table 13-2 *Locations of the Precordial Electrodes*

Lead	Location
V_1	Fourth intercostal space at the right sternal border
V_2	Fourth intercostal space at the left sternal border
V_3	Midway between V_2 and V_4
V_4	Fifth intercostal space at the midclavicular line
V_5	Fifth intercostal space at the anterior axillary line
V_6	Fifth intercostal space at the midaxillary line

Table 13-3 Sensor Lead Placement and a Common Coding System

Lead	Location	Marking Code	Color Code	
			Body	Insert
Standard or bipolar limb leads				
Lead I (RA-LA)	Right arm to left arm	•	Green	Green
Lead II (RA-LL)	Right arm to left leg	••	RA-white, LL-red	RA-gray, LL-red
Lead III (LA-LL)	Left arm to left leg	•••	Black	Gray
Augmented unipolar limb leads				
aVR (LA-LL) RA	RA-midpoint (LA-LL)	–	Green	Green
aVL (RA-LL) LA	LA-midpoint (RA-LL)	– –	RA-white, LL-red	RA-gray, LL-red
aVF (RA-LA) LL	LL-midpoint (RA-LA)	– – –	Black	Gray

(continued)

Table 13-3 (Continued)

Lead	Location	Marking Code	Color Code	
Chest or precordial leads				
V_1	Fourth intercostal space, right sternal border	–•	Brown	Red
V_2	Fourth intercostal space, left sternal border	–••	Brown	Yellow
V_3	Midway between V_2 and V_4	–•••	Brown	Green
V_4	Fifth intercostal space, midclavicular left	–••••	Brown	Blue
V_5	Left anterior axillary fold, horizontal to V_4	–•••••	Brown	Orange
V_6	Left midaxillary, horizontal to V_4 and V_5	–••••••	Brown	Violet

Written Information on an ECG Recording

An ECG recording should contain the following written information:

- The patient's full name
- Date and time of ECG
- Address
- Age (date of birth)
- Sex
- The patient's ID
- Blood pressure
- Height and weight
- The doctor's name
- Medications the patient is taking

Normal Adult ECG

The electrical activity through the heart is displayed in a series of waves and complexes. These waves make up the cardiac cycle. The normal cardiac cycle includes the following waves and complexes:

- P wave—contraction of the atria
- QRS complex—contraction of both ventricles
- T wave—relaxation of both ventricles
- U wave—small upright waveform, sometimes seen after the T wave, but before the next P wave

See Figure 13-1 for the various waves listed above.

Key Focus: P, R, T, and U waves are upward (positive) deflection, and Q and S waves are downward (negative) deflection.

The shape of the various waves on an ECG may be

- Normal
- Wide
- Short
- Tall
- Flat
- Bizarre
- Spiked

Characteristics of ECG waves and complexes are summarized in Table 13-4.

Table 13-4 *Characteristics of Electrocardiogram Waves and Complexes*

Waves and Complexes	Characteristics
P wave	Represents atrial depolarization The normal P is small, upright, and rounded Duration is less than 0.11 seconds
PR interval	Represents AV conduction time Duration is 0.12–0.20 seconds
QRS complex	Represents ventricular depolarization Duration is less than 0.10 seconds Q is the first negative, R is the positive wave, and S is the next negative wave
Q wave	The first downward (negative) deflection, related to the initial phase of depolarization
R wave	The first upward (positive) deflection, representing ventricular depolarization

Table 13-4 *(Continued)*

Waves and Complexes	Characteristics
S wave	The second downward (negative) deflection
QT interval	The time between the start of the Q wave and the end of the T wave
ST segment	Represents early ventricular repolarization
T wave	Represents ventricular repolarization
	The normal T wave is rounded and broad
U wave	Represents late repolarization and is not normally seen
	If present, the U wave follows the T wave
	The U wave may be influenced by low serum potassium level or other metabolic disorder

Artifacts

Artifacts are abnormal signals that do not reflect electrical activity of the heart during the cardiac cycle. The following factors may cause artifacts:

- Patient movement
- Mechanical problems with the ECG machine
- Improper technique

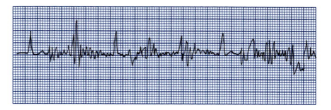

Figure 13-4 *Electrocardiogram artifacts.*

> **Key Focus:** While the medical assistant is taking an ECG, they should ask the patient not to move, cough, or talk. The machine must be away from walls and any electrical wiring or other equipment. The machine must also be regularly checked and maintained for accuracy.

The medical assistant is responsible for obtaining a good-quality ECG without avoidable artifacts. Figure 13-4 shows ECG artifacts. Generally, there are four types of artifacts, as follows:

- Wandering baseline
- Somatic (muscle) tremor
- Alternating current
- Interrupted baseline

> **Key Focus:** If artifacts are seen, unplug any electrical equipment in the area that you are conducting the ECG.

HOLTER MONITOR

The Holter monitor is a portable electrical device that may be worn comfortably for at least 24 hours to record cardiac activity. Holter monitoring is performed without interfering with daily activities. Holter monitors are used when cardiac irregularity has not been determined on a tracing. These monitors are used with a small tape recorder and a patient diary to detect heart irregularities not commonly detected on a standard 12-lead cardiogram. Figure 13-5 shows a digital Holter monitor.

Sensors

The five sensors of the Holter monitor are attached to these locations:

- Third intercostal space, 2 or 3 inches to the right of sternum
- Third intercostal space, 2 or 3 inches to the left of sternum
- Fifth intercostal space at left sternum margin

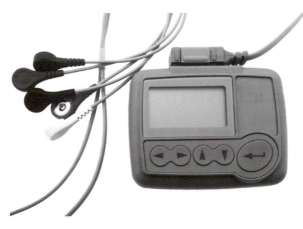

Brittny/Shutterstock

Figure 13-5 *A digital Holter monitor.*

- Sixth intercostal space at right anterior axillary line
- Sixth intercostal space at left anterior axillary line

> **Key Focus:** The five special disposable chest sensors of the Holter monitor are attached more securely than those used in the 12-lead ECG.

MOBILE CARDIAC TELEMETRY

Mobile cardiac telemetry (MCT) allows some patients to have their heart activity monitored and measured over long distances. A device sends data continually to a monitoring facility 24 hours per day. Cardiac-trained nurses interpret the data, allowing real-time monitoring and analysis. Telemetry monitors may have 3, 5, or 12 leads, placed by following manufacturer instructions. Figure 13-6 shows a telemetry monitor known as a "ZIO Patch." Medical assistants must ensure the patient knows how to use the telemetry monitor, and should encourage the patient to call the "help number" to learn how to attach the leads and ask for help if problems occur.

TREADMILL STRESS TEST

The treadmill stress test (or exercise tolerance ECG) may be prescribed to determine a diagnosis and prognosis for heart disorders, chest pain, and cardiac ability after cardiac surgery. As a result of using the treadmill, the additional workload on the patient's myocardium will often be seen as an abnormality on the ECG. Frequent blood pressure readings are taken during close monitoring while the patient is on the treadmill. At the end of the test, the patient must rest while monitoring continues until

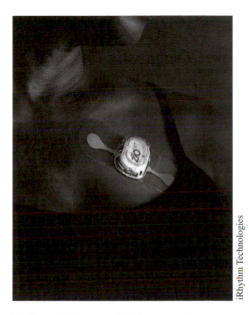

Figure 13-6 *A "ZIO Patch" Telemetry Monitor.*

heart rate and vital signs return to normal. During these tests, electrodes are applied to the torso, with precordial sensors (V_1–V_6) placed as they are in a regular ECG. Arm and leg sensors are instead placed at the midclavicular line on the top of the torso, and on the midclavicular line on the abdomen.

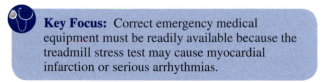

Key Focus: Correct emergency medical equipment must be readily available because the treadmill stress test may cause myocardial infarction or serious arrhythmias.

CHAPTER 14
Diagnostic Imaging

Various techniques exist to visualize internal body structures for diagnoses and treatments. They include

- Radiography (x-rays)
- Magnetic resonance imaging (MRI)
- Ultrasound (or sonography)

RADIOLOGY

Radiology is divided into three specialties:

- Diagnostic radiology
- Radiation therapy
- Nuclear medicine

X-rays

Radiography is the process of taking x-rays, which exhibit the following characteristics:

- Penetrate substances of different densities to varying degrees
- Cause ionization of the substances they penetrate
- Cause fluorescence of certain substances (allowing physicians to visualize structures in motion)
- Travel in a straight line (x-ray beam can be directed at a specific area)
- Can destroy body cells and cancer cells

X-ray Machine Components

- Tube in its barrel-shaped tube housing
- Collimator, mounted on tube housing

- Tube housing with attachments, mounted on tube support or suspended from ceiling
- Radiographic table, upright cassette holder
- Control console, where operator selects exposure setting and makes exposure (in control booth)

COMMON RADIOLOGICAL IMAGING EXAMINATIONS

- Angiography
  - Visualization of a blood vessel
  - Injection of radiopaque material
  - Diagnoses—blood flow, myocardial infarction, stroke, or aneurysm
- Arthrography
  - Image inside of a joint
  - Uses a contrast medium and fluoroscopy
  - Diagnoses—problems in cartilage, tendons, ligaments of knee, hip, shoulder
- Barium enema (lower GI)
  - Outlines colon, rectum on a radiographic image
  - Administration of barium sulfate
  - Diagnoses—polyps, ulcers, diverticulosis, or tumors
- Barium swallow (upper GI series)
  - Looks at esophagus, stomach, duodenum, small intestine
  - Patient drinks a barium solution
  - Diagnoses—ulcers, polyps, tumors, diverticulosis, or motility problems
- Cholangiography
  - X-ray during gallbladder surgery
  - Injection of a contrast medium
  - Evaluates function of the bile ducts
- Cholecystography
  - Radiological exam of gallbladder

- X-ray—after patient ingests contrast medium
- Diagnoses—bile duct obstructions, gallstones
- Computed tomography (CT)
  - Combines radiography with computer analysis of tissue density
  - Produces a three-dimensional, cross-sectional view of an area of the body
  - Diagnoses—lesions in areas like the brain, liver, gallbladder, spleen
- Fluoroscopy
  - Visually examining a body area or function of an organ using a fluoroscope
  - Produces moving image that can be filmed using x-rays, for permanent record
- Intravenous pyelography (IVP)
  - X-rays of kidneys, ureters, and bladder
  - Contrast medium with iodine injected into vein
  - Diagnoses—urinary system abnormalities or trauma to the urinary system
- Kidneys, ureters, and bladder (KUB) radiography—x-rays abdomen, pelvis to assess size, shape, location, diseases of organs of urinary tract and to detect kidney stones, intrauterine devices (IUDs), foreign objects.
- MRI—powerful magnetic field produces an image of internal tissues, organs, and structures
- Mammography
  - X-ray examination of the breasts
  - Diagnoses—various tumors
- Myelography
  - Fluoroscopic procedure of spinal cord
  - Lumbar puncture removes some cerebrospinal fluid and a contrast medium is instilled
  - Diagnoses—compression of spinal cord, herniated disks, tumors, cysts, or spinal stenosis

- Nuclear medicine (radionuclide imaging)—radioactive isotopes for diagnosis and treatment of disease
- Radiation therapy—cancer treatment that uses x-rays to damage and destroy cancer cells
- Retrograde pyelogram
  - Radiopaque material injected through a urinary catheter into ureters and kidney
  - Evaluates function of ureters, bladder, and urethra
- Stereoscopy
  - X-ray procedure using a specially designed microscope
  - Diagnoses—fractures, tumors, or increased pressure within the skull
- Thermography
  - Infrared camera takes photographs of variations in skin temperature
  - Dark = cool areas; light = warm areas
  - Diagnoses—breast tumors, breast abscesses, and fibrocystic breast disease
- Ultrasound (sonography)
  - Uses high-frequency sound waves to image internal structures
  - Often used for fetal monitoring
  - Diagnoses—gallstones, tumors, heart defects
- Xeroradiography
  - X-rays developed with powder toner
  - Image is processed on specially treated xerographic paper
  - Diagnoses—breast cancer, abscesses, or tissue calcifications

Diagnostic Imaging

Key Focus: Among the most common fluoroscopic examinations are studies of the lower and upper gastrointestinal tract.

PREPARING THE PATIENT

The medical assistant is responsible for the following:

- Schedule procedure ordered
- Patient education
- Explain preparations before procedure
- Inform patient about duration of procedure
- Give written instructions to the patient
- Provide post-procedure instructions
- Inform patient when to expect results

Table 14-1 describes x-ray procedures that require special preparations.

Table 14-1 *X-ray Procedures That Require Special Preparations*

Procedure	Preparation
Angiogram	Patient should have no breakfast if it is a morning examination; no lunch if afternoon examination. Cerebral angiograms: 2–3 hours; coronary angiograms: 20–30 minutes. Most other types of angiograms take about 1 hour
Barium enema (lower GI)	Enemas used until bowel return is clear on evening before exam. A rectal suppository may be ordered in morning (or a cathartic such as 2 ounces of castor oil or citrate of magnesia at 4 P.M. the day before x-ray); clear liquids, Jell-O for evening meal; nothing by mouth (NPO) after midnight

Procedure	Preparation
Barium swallow (upper GI)	NPO after midnight
Cholecystogram (GB series)	A light evening meal of nonfatty foods (fruits, vegetables without butter or oil) evening before x-ray; prescribed gallbladder tablets taken with water after evening meal; NPO except for water until x-ray the following day
Computerized tomography (CT)	NPO for 4 hours prior to x-ray if a contrast medium is to be used
Intravenous cholangiogram (x-ray of the biliary tree)	NPO. A clear liquid diet the day before the test
Intravenous pyelogram (IVP)	Three oral bisacodyl (Dulcolax) tablets or 2 ounces of castor oil at 4 P.M. the day prior to the x-ray; eat a light evening meal; NPO after midnight
Myelogram (x-ray spine, spinal cord, and spinal structures)	NPO for 8 hours prior to procedure. The procedure itself takes about 1 hour
Retrograde pyelogram	Enemas, laxatives evening prior to x-ray; NPO for 8 hours before procedure
Ultrasound	A full bladder or laxatives may be required for some ultrasounds

Diagnostic Imaging

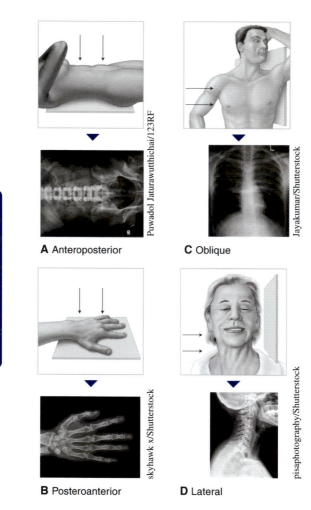

A Anteroposterior

C Oblique

B Posteroanterior

D Lateral

Puwadol Jaturawutthichai/123RF

Jayakumar/Shutterstock

skyhawk x/Shutterstock

pisaphotography/Shutterstock

Figure 14-1 *Common x-ray positions and images.*

Diagnostic Imaging

Various Positions

The position determines the image result of the x-ray. Figure 14-1 shows examples of the most common x-ray positions and the images they produce.

The position of the patient is critical for an accurate x-ray. Table 14-2 lists radiology positions.

Table 14-2 *Radiology Positions*

Position	Description
Anteroposterior (AP)	X-ray beam directed from front to back. Patient may be standing or supine. Patient's front faces x-ray equipment; patient's back near the film plate
Axial	X-ray tube angled to direct a ray along axis of body or body part. In cephalad angulation, x-ray beam is directed at an angle from the feet toward the head. In caudad angulation, the x-ray beam is directed from the head toward the feet
Lateral	X-ray beam directed toward one side of body. In right lateral (RL) position, patient's right side is near film plate, and left side is near x-ray equipment. In a left lateral (LL) position, the patient's left side is near the film plate

(continued)

Table 14-2 (*Continued*)

Position	Description
Oblique	The patient is turned at an angle to the film plate so that the x-ray beam can be directed at areas that would be hidden on an AP, PA, or lateral x-ray
Posteroanterior (PA)	X-ray beam directed from back to front. Patient standing upright, back will face x-ray equipment. Patient's front is near film plate

PROCEDURE 14-1 *Assisting with an X-ray Examination*

Most common routine plain films are performed in physicians' offices by medical assistants and include extremities, chest, spine. In some states, medical assistants can't perform radiology. Equipment and supplies needed:

- Patient identification card to imprint radiographs
- X-ray machine (see Figure 14-2 on student resources website)
- X-ray cassettes, loaded with film
- Accessory items such as lead patient shields
- X-ray darkroom with automatic processor
- Dosimeter badges

Method

1. Check the x-ray examination order.
2. Check the necessary x-ray equipment.

3. Confirm the identity of the patient.
4. Explain the procedure to the patient.
5. Place the x-ray cassette correctly.
6. Make sure that the patient has removed all jewelry and metal objects as needed for the procedure.
7. Position and drape the patient correctly.
8. Align the x-ray tube and the cassette at the proper distance and set the controls.
9. Ask the patient to hold their breath as necessary.
10. Stand behind a lead shield during the exposure.
11. In darkroom, remove film from cassette, identify the film, and process the film in the automatic processor.
12. Instruct the patient to dress if the x-rays are satisfactory.
13. Label the x-rays and place them in the proper envelope according to office procedures.
14. Document the procedure appropriately.

Key Focus: X-ray personnel are not exposed to any significant amount of radiation when standing well behind protective lead barrier of control booth.

RADIATION THERAPY TECHNIQUES

The two methods of administering radiation include

• External radiation therapy (ERT)—administration of calculated amounts of radiation from a machine positioned at a certain distance from a tumor site. A tattoo or marker is placed on the patient at the exact site. A computer calculates the best dosage to destroy the greatest number of malignant cells while causing the lowest amount of damage to surrounding cells. Treatments may be needed over weeks or months.

- Internal radiation therapy (IRT)—administered in two forms: *sealed* or *unsealed* radiation:
  - Sealed radiation—implanting sealed containers of radioactive material near the tumor. Examples: cesium-137, cobalt-60, and radium, sealed in small gold seeds or containers.
  - Unsealed radiation—liquid form of a radioactive substance, by mouth, via blood stream, or by instillation into body cavity. Examples: gold-198, phosphorus-32, and radioactive iodine-131.

Radiation therapy usually causes no disfigurement. Symptoms vary, lasting 3 to 6 weeks, and may include

- Hair loss
- Skin changes
- Nausea
- Diarrhea
- Irritation of mucous membranes of the mouth, throat, bladder, or vagina
- Chromosomal changes

RADIATION SAFETY

Two systems are used to measure radiation and the radiation dose, which include

- The conventional (British) system—the most commonly used in the United States
- The international system

Key Focus: Occupational exposure to x-rays increases when assisting with fluoroscopic procedures or when using mobile x-ray equipment.

Personnel Monitoring

Devices for monitoring radiation exposure to personnel are called dosimeters. They should be worn in the region of the collar, outside the lead apron (see Figure 14-3).

Maintaining Personnel Safety

- Film badges worn at all times on outer clothing without being concealed by gowns or lead shields.
- Film badges must be submitted regularly (usually weekly) to evaluate radiation exposure levels.
- Lead shields should be used to separate personnel from the x-ray equipment while in use.
- The x-ray room should be lead lined.
- The x-ray room door should be closed when the equipment is in use, with a lighted sign or display that indicates when the equipment is operating.
- Only essential personnel should be in the x-ray room during procedures.
- Radiation leakage should be regularly checked for during equipment inspections.

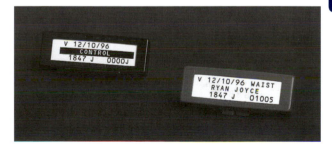

Figure 14-3 *Dosimeter.*

- Patients should only be held or positioned during radiologic procedures by equipment—never by the personnel conducting the procedure.
- Personnel who must be in x-ray room with patients should wear lead aprons, lead-lined rubber gloves.
- Personnel should always face patient during procedures, keeping lead apron between them and the patient.
- Personnel are periodically blood tested to determine abnormalities that exist due to radiation exposure.

Maintaining Patient Safety

- The patient should be questioned about any recent x-ray procedures or possible exposure to x-rays due to any work-related activities.
- Female patients should be asked whether they are pregnant; if so, this must be reported to physician before x-ray procedure is conducted; a release (and pregnancy test) should be obtained to prevent liability.
- Female patients should be especially advised of potential radiation risks.
- A lead shield should be placed over all abdominal and reproductive organs of the patient.
- Patients must be positioned with care to obtain accurate image and avoid need for re-exposure to radiation.
- Personnel fully trained and instructed, with proper state authorization, may do any x-ray procedure.

Visit www.pearsonhighered.com/healthprofessionsresources to access figures and tables available on the student resources website. Click on view all resources and select Medical Assisting from the choice of disciplines. Find this book and you can see all respective tables and figures.

SECTION IV
Laboratory Procedures

Laboratory
Procedures

CHAPTER 15
Diagnostic Phlebotomy and Hematology

Medical assistants are trained to perform phlebotomy and may have to collect blood samples as part of their regular work activities. Phlebotomy is usually performed to diagnose and monitor a patient's condition. The most common methods of obtaining blood are

- Venipuncture
- Capillary puncture

Venipuncture is performed in a variety of locations on the body. The upper extremities are the easiest and safest sites from which to collect blood (see Figure 15-1).

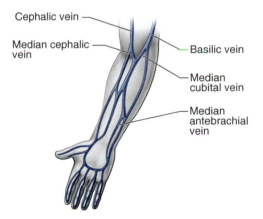

Cephalic vein

Median cephalic vein

Basilic vein

Median cubital vein

Median antebrachial vein

Figure 15-1 *Anatomy of an arm for venipuncture.*

PROCEDURE 15-1 *Venipuncture*

Routine venipuncture is a common type of blood collection and is regularly done in the physician's office using the following equipment and supplies:

- Gloves
- Alcohol swabs
- Gauze pads
- Evacuated, stoppered tubes
- Evacuated tube holders
- Double-pointed safety needles
- Butterfly systems
- Needle and syringe systems
- Lancets
- Microtainer tubes
- Tourniquet
- Nonallergenic bandages
- Venipuncture chair
- Smelling salts
- Biohazard sharps container

Method

The most common method of venipuncture is the evacuated tube method, which requires the following steps:

1. Review requisition slip.
2. Identify the patient.
3. Gather supplies.
4. Perform hand hygiene and apply gloves.
5. Explain the procedure to the patient.
6. Apply tourniquet, select vein, and release tourniquet.

7. Cleanse site and reapply tourniquet.
8. Remove cap from needle and examine needle.
9. Anchor vein and insert needle at a 15°–30° angle.
10. Keep the bevel up.
11. Push tube completely into adapter and make sure that you do not move the needle after it enters the vein.
12. Remove tube after it is completely filled and insert next tube if required.
13. Gently invert tubes.
14. Release tourniquet as last tube is filled.
15. Remove needle and place gauze over puncture site.
16. Dispose of the needle in a biohazard sharps container and label the tubes.
17. Bandage patient's arm.
18. Dispose of used supplies.
19. Remove gloves, wash hands, and transport specimens.

Figure 15-2 demonstrates the venipuncture procedure.

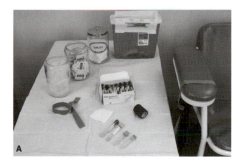

Figure 15-2 *Venipuncture procedure.* (*Continued*)

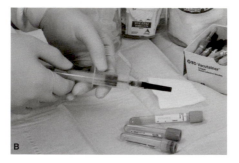

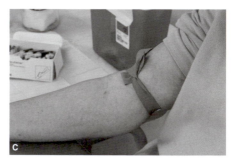

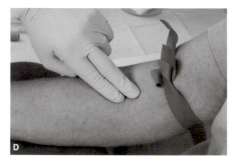

Figure 15-2 (*Continued*)

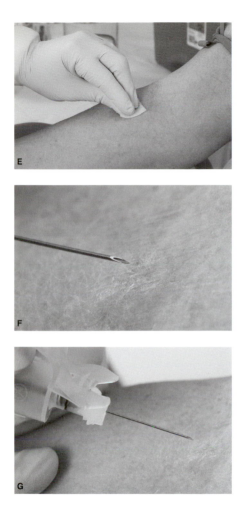

Figure 15-2 (*Continued*)

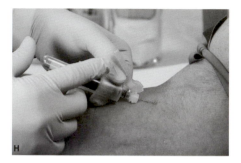

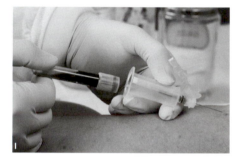

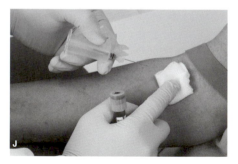

Figure 15-2 (*Continued*)

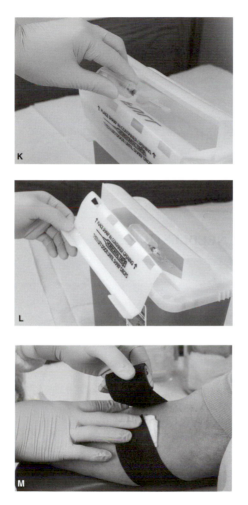

Figure 15-2 (*Continued*)

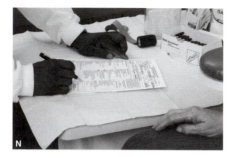

Figure 15-2 (*Continued*)

ACCIDENTAL NEEDLESTICK

The Occupational Safety and Health Act's (OSHA) Bloodborne Pathogens standards suggest follow-up procedures for healthcare workers who are accidentally stuck with potentially contaminated needles:

- The supervising physician should be notified immediately.
- Proper testing and prophylactic treatment must be initiated immediately.
- The employer is responsible for medical evaluation and treatment of any employee.
- The employer should seek to find reasons for the occurrence of a needlestick and to determine whether additional training may be required to prevent such incident in the future.
- All contaminated needlestick incidents must be recorded in a written report.

STANDARD PRECAUTIONS

Standard precautions (by the Centers for Disease Control and Prevention [CDC]) must be utilized when dealing with any infectious materials. All materials that may be biohazards must be labeled with biohazard labels.

Many diseases can be transmitted by poor techniques in the healthcare facility. Standard precautions apply to many body substances, including

- Blood
- Semen
- Cerebrospinal fluid
- Pleural fluid
- Synovial fluid
- Vaginal secretions
- Any other body fluids

Healthcare employers and employees must assume that all human body fluids may be infected with bloodborne pathogens and handle them using standard precautions. These precautions should also be used in dealing with

- Feces
- Nasal secretions
- Sputum
- Breast milk
- Tears
- Saliva
- Urine
- Vomitus
- Broken skin
- Mucous membranes that line the mouth, nose, or other body cavities

STOPPERED TUBES

To perform venipuncture, you need to select specific Vacutainer colors for different tests, with additive. Table 15-1 lists common stoppers and additives, and their laboratory uses in adults and children.

Table 15-1 *Common Stopper Colors and Additives*

Stopper Color	Additives	Tests
Red	None	Chemistry, blood bank, serology/immunology
Light blue	Sodium citrate	Coagulation studies
Red and gray mottled (Gold Hemogard)	Clot activator/silica particles	Routine blood donor screening and infectious disease testing
Green	Heparin	Electrolyte studies, arterial blood gases
Lavender	Ethylenediamine tetraacetic acid (EDTA) (anticoagulant)	Hematology and blood chemistries
Gray	Potassium oxalate or sodium fluoride (anticoagulant)	Blood glucose
Yellow	Sodium polyanethol sulfonate (SPS)	Blood cultures

PROCEDURE 15-2 *Butterfly Method*

In some cases, you must obtain a venous sample accurately by using butterfly method from a small vein on the hand, or a vein that is compromised (as in elderly patients) (see Figure 15-3) by using the following:

- Gloves
- Alcohol pads
- Gauze pads

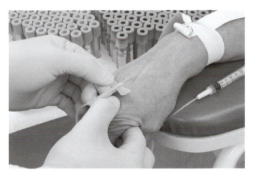

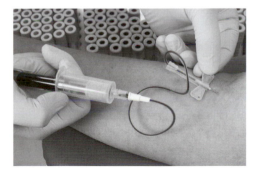

Figure 15-3 *The butterfly method.*

- Tourniquet
- Butterfly needle set
- Luer-Lok syringe or evacuated tube holder
- Appropriate pediatric tubes arranged in the order of the draw
- Sharps disposal container
- Nonallergenic bandage
- Permanent marking pen

Method

1. Check the laboratory requisition for the procedure to be performed.
2. Gather the appropriate tubes needed for the test(s), as well as all other required supplies.
3. Wash hands and put on protective equipment.
4. Prepare the patient, placing them in a sitting position with the arm supported, in a slightly downward position.
5. Remove butterfly device from the package, stretching it slightly, which helps keep the tube from recoiling.
6. Attach the butterfly device to the syringe, or to an evacuated tube holder.
7. Seat the first tube into the evacuated tube holder.
8. Apply the tourniquet to the patient's wrist near the wrist bone.
9. Hold the patient's hand with your fingers lower than their wrist.
10. Select a vein and cleanse the site to be pierced.
11. Pull the patient's skin taut over their knuckles by using your thumb.
12. Align needle with the vein at a 10°–15° angle (the bevel should be up).
13. Insert needle gently by threading it up the lumen of the vein so that it will not twist out of the vein.

14. Push the blood collecting tube onto the end of the holder (or draw blood into the syringe).
15. Release tourniquet when the blood appears inside the tube.
16. Keep the tube and holder always in a downward position, allowing the tube to fill from the bottom up.
17. Place a pad of gauze over the puncture site and gently remove the needle.
18. Have the patient apply direct pressure on the puncture site using the gauze pad, and then have them elevate their arm, which helps stop bleeding.
19. Invert the blood collecting tube to mix anticoagulants and blood; do this gently, without shaking or vigorously mixing the contents (to avoid hemolysis).
20. Label the tube with the patient's name, date, and time of collection.
21. Check the puncture site for any bleeding and apply a hypoallergenic bandage.
22. Remove gloves and face protection, clean the work area, and wash your hands.
23. Complete the laboratory requisition form and route it to the proper location.
24. Record the procedure in the patient's record.

PROCEDURE 15-3 *Capillary Puncture*

Capillaries connect small arterioles to small venules. Capillary (dermal) puncture is performed when small amounts of blood are required, or when a patient's condition makes venipuncture difficult. Capillary puncture is indicated for

- Pediatric patients (under 2 years of age)

- Obese patients
- Elderly patients
- Patients who have had a mastectomy
- Patients who are at risk for venous thrombosis
- Patients who are receiving intravenous therapy
- Patients who have burns or scars in venipuncture sites
- Patients who are severely dehydrated
- Patients who require frequent glucose monitoring
- When venous blood and capillary blood are not identical (e.g., hemoglobin and glucose values are higher in capillary blood, while potassium, calcium, and total protein are higher in venous blood)

The following equipment and supplies are required:

- Lancet
- Automatic devices—which deliver a quick puncture to a predetermined depth
- Microsample containers with color codings
- Alcohol swabs
- Sterile gauze
- Nonallergenic tape

Site of Selection

The usual puncture sites for adults and children are as follows:

- The ring finger at the tip and slightly to the side of the finger
- The middle finger at the tip and slightly to the side of the finger
- The heel (for infants younger than 1 year, the medial or lateral surfaces of the heel are used)
- Outer edge of the ear lobe

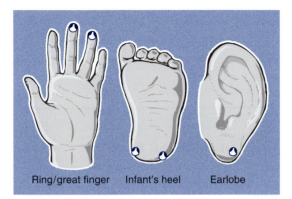

Figure 15-4 *Capillary puncture sites.*

Figure 15-4 shows the common capillary puncture sites.

Method

1. Using the physician's requisition, assemble all required materials.
2. Select a puncture site for the procedure.
3. Gently rub the finger along the sites to be punctured; for capillary puncture of the heel, wrap it with warm towels prior to the puncture. If the patient's hands are cold, run warm water over them to facilitate blood flow.
4. Grasp the patient's finger firmly, or their heel if that site is to be used.
5. Hold the lancet at a right angle and make the puncture.
6. Wipe away the first drop of blood that escapes the puncture site.
7. Apply pressure by lightly squeezing the site to cause the blood to flow freely.

8. Collect blood samples as required.
9. Make sure that the patient's bleeding is under control.
10. If the patient is a child under 2 years of age, do not place bandages anywhere on them, as bandages could become a choking hazard.
11. Bandage the puncture site if the patient is of appropriate age.

ORDER OF DRAWING BLOOD

Medical assistants must understand the importance of drawing blood in the correct order.

- Blood culture tubes
- Light blue stopper
- Red stopper (nonadditive) or SST (red/gray or gold)—serum separator tubes
- Green stopper
- Purple stopper
- Gray stopper

HEMATOLOGY

A variety of hematological tests may be performed in the clinical laboratory.

Key Focus: Medical assistants are only allowed to perform blood tests allowed under Clinical Laboratory Improvement Amendments (CLIA) of 1988. Examination of white blood cells under microscope for differential test should be done by a physician, not an M.A.

White and Red Blood Cell Counts

A complete blood count (CBC) includes the following tests:

- Red blood (cell) count—total RBCs in a specimen, and red cell morphology
- White blood (cell) count—total WBCs in a specimen
- Differential WBC count—percentage of basophils, eosinophils, neutrophils, lymphocytes, and monocytes in the first 100 leukocytes of a specimen
- Platelet count (automated)—platelets in a specimen, or an estimate, indicating whether number of platelets is adequate
- Hematocrit determination—how much of specimen volume (in %) is made up of RBCs after being spun in a centrifuge
- Hemoglobin determination—amount of hemoglobin by weight, per volume, in the specimen

Differential cell counts may be performed by medical assistants, using blood smear slides that are stained to obtain a manual differential cell count. A polychromatic (multicolored) stain such as Wright's stain is often used, utilizing blue and red-orange dyes. Staining characteristics of each type of WBC are as follows:

- Basophils—purple nucleus, light purple cytoplasm that contains large, blue-black granules
- Eosinophils—purple nucleus, bright orange granules in pink cytoplasm
- Neutrophils—dark purple nucleus, pale pink cytoplasm with fine pink or lavender granules
- Lymphocytes—large, dark purple nucleus surrounded by small amount of blue cytoplasm
- Monocytes—largest WBC, has gray-blue cytoplasm

WBC and RBC counts may be performed by the following methods:

- Manually, by using a microscope
- Automated blood analyzer

Both require small blood samples, to be diluted in *unopettes* (prefilled reservoirs with a premeasured diluting fluid unit). Manually, WBC or RBC counts are obtained by using a hemocytometer—a slide-counting chamber that allows cells to be counted under a microscope. Follow instructions to ensure the validity of the result.

Key Focus: The manual method is less accurate and not as reliable as the automated blood analyzer.

PROCEDURE 15-4 *Differential White Blood Cell Counts*

These tests may be done by using a microscope with a bright light and 100×magnification, as well as an oil immersion slide using the following equipment and supplies:

- Gloves
- Clean glass slides
- Whole blood (EDTA)
- Eye dropper
- Wright's stain
- Distilled water
- Permanent ink pen
- Biohazard container

PROCEDURE 15-5 *Hemoglobin Measurement*

Hemoglobin can be measured either by an automated blood analyzer or manually by using a hemoglobinometer. Normal hemoglobin values are listed in Table 15-2. Equipment and supplies needed are

- Gloves
- Alcohol pads
- Gauze pads
- Sterile lancet
- Glass slide chamber
- Hemoglobinometer
- Hemolysis applicator (plastic or wooden)
- Biohazard sharps container

Method

1. Obtain capillary blood by using a sterile lancet.
2. Pull the glass chamber out of the hemoglobinometer and position the lower part of the slide so that it is slightly offset.
3. Place a large drop of capillary blood onto the slide.
4. Apply a dry gauze on the puncture and use a bandage.

Table 15-2 *Normal Hemoglobin Values by Age or Sex*

Individual	Normal Range (g/dL)
Newborn	17–23
Age 3 months	9–14
Age 10 months	12–14.5
Adult male	13–18
Adult female	12–16

5. Mix blood with a hemolysis applicator until the blood becomes clear.
6. Push the glass chamber into the clip and place into the slot on the left side of the hemoglobinometer.
7. Hold the hemoglobinometer at eye level and turn on the light.
8. Look into the instrument to see a split green field.
9. Look at the meter until a matching green field occurs.
10. Read the hemoglobin value at the top scale. The results are read as grams of hemoglobin per 100 mL of blood (g/dL).

PROCEDURE 15-6 *Hematocrit Measurement*

The hematocrit (packed RBC volume) is the ratio of the volume of packed RBCs to that of the whole-blood specimen. Packed RBC volume is expressed as a percentage of the whole specimen. Equipment and supplies needed are

- Gloves
- Capillary tubes
- Sealing clay
- Microhematocrit
- Centrifuge
- Whole blood
- Hematocrit (Hct) card
- Biohazard sharps container

Method

1. Gather supplies.
2. Fill two capillary tubes 3/4 full.
3. Seal one end with the sealing clay.
4. Place capillary tubes in the centrifuge with the sealed ends against the rubber gasket.
5. Spin for 3–5 minutes at 10,000 rpm.

Table 15-3 *Normal Hematocrit Values by Age or Sex*

Individual	Normal Range (%)
Newborn	45–60
1-year-old child	27–44
Adult male	40–55
Adult female	36–46

6. Remove tubes immediately after the centrifuge stops.
7. Determine results. Use the Hct card by placing the sealing clay just below the zero line on both tubes directly below the buffy coat. Add the results together and divide by 2.
8. Normal hematocrit values are summarized in Table 15-3.

RBC Indices

- Mean corpuscular volume (MCV)
  - Measures the size of RBCs
  - Calculated by dividing the hematocrit by the number of RBCs per liter
- Mean corpuscular hemoglobin (MCH)
  - Average mass of hemoglobin found in each RBC
  - Calculated by dividing the total mass of hemoglobin by the RBC count
- Mean corpuscular hemoglobin concentration (MCHC)
  - Amount of the concentration of hemoglobin in the cells
  - Calculated by dividing the hemoglobin by the hematocrit

Key Focus: The most important index for classification of anemias is MCV.

PROCEDURE 15-7 *Erythrocyte Sedimentation Rate*

The erythrocyte sedimentation rate (ESR) measures the rate at which RBCs settle at the bottom of a tube. This test is used as a general indication of inflammation. The following equipment and supplies are needed:

- Gloves
- Whole blood (EDTA)
- Wintrobe tube
- Wintrobe rack
- Permanent ink pen
- Biohazard sharps container

Method

1. Assemble equipment.
2. Obtain a whole-blood sample using a purple topped tube.
3. Slowly fill the Wintrobe tube with blood, avoiding air bubbles.
4. Adjust the meniscus of the specimen to the zero line at the top of the tube.
5. Maintain the tube in an upright vertical position for 1 hour.
6. After 1 hour, record the number of RBCs that settle.
7. Read the ESR on the same side of the tube's zero line, at the top.

PROCEDURE 15-8 *Bleeding Time*

This test evaluates clotting disorders and determines effectiveness of coagulation therapy. Equipment needed are

- Gloves

- Alcohol pads
- Blood pressure cuff
- Autolet device
- Filter paper
- Stopwatch
- Bandage

Method

1. Position the patient so that the arm is extended.
2. Select the inner aspect of the arm several inches below the antecubital area.
3. Apply the pressure cuff and set it at 40 mmHg for the length of the test.
4. Make an incision 1 mm in depth on the cleaned skin surface with the Autolet.
5. At 30-second intervals, bring the filter paper near the edge of the wound to draw off some of the accumulating blood.
6. Change the area of absorption on the filter paper each time. Avoid touching the wound with the filter paper.
7. When the blood flow stops, the test is completed. Stop the watch and remove the pressure cuff.

CHEMICAL TESTS

Blood chemistry analysis examines several dozen chemicals found in the blood. Complex testing must follow strict CLIA '88 regulations, increasing administrative work and the need for highly trained personnel. Automated equipment for analyzing blood chemistry is now more available, less expensive, and easier to operate than in the past.

Blood Glucose Monitoring

Blood glucose monitoring is often performed by medical assistants, and even by patients themselves. Blood is collected on reagent strips that change color, based on glucose levels in the blood. Levels are determined by comparing the color on the strip with color guides that are packaged with the strips, or by using a handheld reading device.

Hemoglobin A1c

The hemoglobin A1c test measures the amount of glycosylated hemoglobin (which has glycosyl groups attached to it) in the blood. Elevated blood glucose levels cause glucose molecules to bind with hemoglobin to form hemoglobin A1c (HgbA1c), which remains in RBC throughout their life (90 to 120 days).

Cholesterol Test

Blood cholesterol tests are routinely performed with automated devices, in laboratories, and by patients to use at home. These devices analyze blood chemicals (glucose, HDL cholesterol, total cholesterol, and triglycerides).

Serological Tests

Serological tests are used to detect specific substances in blood. *"Serological test"* and *"immunoassay"* refer to introduction of antigens or antibodies and detection of related reactions. Serological tests detect the presence of

- Disease antibodies
- Drugs
- Hormones
- Vitamins

Serological tests are also used to determine blood type, and to test urine and other body fluids.

CHAPTER 16
Microbiology

The study of microorganisms is called microbiology. Most microbes are not pathogenic (only 1–2% cause diseases). Microbiology today is a complex field and encompasses the following studies:

- Bacteriology
- Microbacteriology
- Virology
- Mycology
- Parasitology

Key Focus: Microbacteriology and virology testing may be limited or not performed at all in smaller institutions.

CLASSIFICATIONS OF MICROORGANISMS

Microorganism classifications are shown in Table 16-1 (see on student resources website).

Key Focus: Unusual bacteria that fall between the size range of viruses and typical pathogenic bacteria include the genera *Chlamydia*, *Mycoplasma*, and *Rickettsia*. Classification of these organisms has posed a challenge to microbiologists.

Indirect methods include
- Antibody reactions
- DNA probes
- Immunofluorescence

Culturing Media

Some bacteria are required to be cultured because they are not easily seen on a direct smear.

- Basic media: used for routine purposes
- Enriched media: have additives to encourage the growth of fastidious organisms
- Carbohydrate-metabolism media: have a specific carbohydrate and indicator added
- Differential media: contain additives that permit visual differentiation of bacteria; an example is MacConkey medium that contains lactose
- Transport media: protect pathogens during transport; may have charcoal, absorbs bacterial wastes

PROCEDURE 16-1 *Performing a Gram Stain*

Gram staining of microorganisms uses a violet-colored solution, then an iodine solution; decolorized with alcohol or acetone solution; counterstained with safranin. Gram stain divides most bacteria into Gram positives or negatives.

The following equipment and supplies are needed:

- Gram stain kit with decolorizer
- Culture specimen
- Slides
- Bunsen burner or methanol
- Staining rack
- Water wash bottle

- Water
- Immersion oil
- Gloves
- Slide stand
- Stopwatch
- Paper towels
- Hazardous waste container

Method

1. Perform hand hygiene and apply gloves.
2. Assemble equipment.
3. Make a smear, label it, and air dry the smear side facing upward.
4. Pour crystal violet solution all over the slide.
5. Rinse the slide with water.
6. Pour Gram's iodine stain all over the slide and wait for 1 minute.
7. Rinse the slide with water.
8. Gently pour decolorizer with alcohol or acetone all over the slide for 15 seconds.
9. Rinse the slide with water.
10. Pour safranin stain all over the slide for 30 seconds.
11. Rinse the slide with water.
12. Stand the slide on end on a paper towel so that it can air dry (see Figure 16-1 on student resources website).

COLLECTING SPECIMENS

Proper specimen collection is essential. Incorrect procedures could cause a contaminated or altered specimen of

- Blood
- Cerebrospinal fluid (CSF)—always treated as a Stat procedure

- Stool—waste product from bowel may be tested for bacterial, parasitic, protozoan infections; or for presence of occult blood, and for excessive amounts of fat (steatorrhea)
- Throat—the most frequently requested specimens in the medical office
- Nasal secretions—care taken to label the swabs "left" and "right," to determine from which nostril the specimen was taken
- Sputum—the mucus substance expelled by coughing or clearing the bronchi
- Urine—see Chapter 17
- Wound specimens—sterile swabs used for specimens from a wound or abscess

Gathering Information

The following information should be provided:

- Patient's information (name, address, and telephone number)
- Identification number (to be sure that you have the right patient)
- Gender
- Age
- Insurance information
- Test requested
- Medication the patient is currently receiving
- Diagnosis, if available
- Physician's information (name, address, and telephone number)

Key Focus: Specimens are rejected by outside laboratories if the label or requisition information is incomplete.

Collection Devices

The following devices or equipment are necessary in the collection of specimens:

- Sterile swabs
- Culture tubes
- Specimen collection containers

Specimen Preservation

Specimens should be obtained before beginning any treatment with antibiotics. Essential steps include

- Deliver specimens to the laboratory immediately
- Certain specimens, except blood and cerebrospinal fluid, can be stored in a refrigerator for several hours
- Isolated specimens of *Neisseria gonorrhoeae* must be submitted on appropriate Martin-Lewis or Neigon agar isolation plates; inoculated plates should not be refrigerated
- Stool specimens being examined for ova or parasites must be preserved in a formalin fixative and PVA (or equivalent) immediately after being collected
- For mycobacterial (TB) culture, three sputum specimens must be collected for acid-fast smears and culture, in 8- to 24-hour intervals
- For blood culture, two to three separate sets must be drawn, within a 24-hour period
- For fever of unknown origin (FUO), two separate sets are drawn initially, then two on next day

CULTURE MEDIA

Once a specimen has been obtained, it must be inoculated onto a medium that will increase the growth of the microorganism. Media may inhibit or encourage the growth of certain microorganisms. Table 16-9 (see on student resources website) shows common culture media and isolations.

Inoculating Media

Pathogens are identified by growing cultures, which are the propagation of microorganisms, taken from a specimen. Colonies of bacteria can be grown only on certain media (see Table 16-9 on student resources website).

Sensitivity Testing

Once the pathogenic organism on the culture is identified, a petri dish with Mueller–Hinton agar and antibiotic disks are used to determine which antibiotics will be effective at killing these bacteria.

- The Mueller–Hinton agar is inoculated with the pure culture specimen in overlapping strokes, and the antibiotic disks are placed in a circle on top of the inoculated agar.
- These are then placed in an incubator for 24 hours. After the most effective antibiotic is identified, the patient is started on drug therapy.

Direct Examination

Two methods are used to prepare a specimen:
- Direct smear
- Wet mount preparation

PROCEDURE 16-2 *Direct Smear*

A direct smear may be from a swab of a specimen or from a colony on a culture plate. Steps include
- Perform hand hygiene and apply gloves.
- Assemble equipment.

- Label a clean slide with the patient's name, date, and type of specimen.
- Inoculate slide by transferring the specimen to slide by rolling the swab over the slide.
- Place a drop of sterile saline on the slide.
- After flaming a needle or loop, pick up the material from one type of colony.
- Place in saline and spread gently over 2/3 of the slide.
- Allow the slide to air dry for 20–30 minutes.
- Hold the slide with thumb forceps and pass the slide over a Bunsen burner flame—this heat "fixes" the specimen to the slide.
- Let the slide cool.
- The slide is then ready to be stained.

PROCEDURE 16-3 *Wet Mount Preparation*

Wet mount preparation involves taking a sample either from a colony or directly from a patient specimen, placing it on a frosted slide, and adding a drop of sterile normal saline and a cover slip.

Method

1. Wash hands and apply gloves.
2. Label a dry slide with the patient's name and date.
3. Inoculate the dry slide by rolling a swab containing a specimen across the surface.
4. Place a drop of saline solution on top of the specimen.
5. Place a cover slip on top of the smeared slide.

Key Focus: A wet mount for fungus is performed using potassium hydroxide (KOH), because fungus is often difficult to see on direct preparation.

PROCEDURES PERFORMED IN THE PHYSICIAN'S OFFICE LABORATORY

In the physician's office, you most likely are involved in patient education, collection of specimens from clients, and performing certain diagnostic tests such as throat cultures and rapid strep tests.

Key Focus: The physician or lab specialist should examine the slide, document observations, perform special stains to enhance characteristics, then remove and dispose of slide.

Microbiology

PROCEDURE 16-4 *Throat Culture of Streptococcus pyogenes*

For inoculating a blood agar plate for culture of *Streptococcus pyogenes*, you will need

- Blood agar plate
- Bacitracin disk or strep A disk
- Incinerator
- Inoculating loop
- Permanent marker
- Swab from patient's throat
- Forceps
- Incubator

Method

1. Wash hands.
2. Put on gloves and apply face protection.
3. Roll the swab down the middle of the top half of the plate, then use the swab to streak the same half of the plate.

4. Sterilize the loop in the Bacti-Cinerator and allow it to cool.
5. Streak for isolation of colonies in the third and fourth quadrants, using the loop.
6. Sterilize the forceps and remove one disk from the vial. Place the disk on the agar in the first quadrant and sterilize the forceps again.
7. Label the agar side of the plate, using a permanent marker, with the patient's name, identification number, and the date.
8. Place the plate in the incubator, with the agar side of the plate on the top.
9. Incubate for 24 hours and then examine.
10. Clean the work area.
11. Dispose of all biohazard wastes.
12. Remove your gloves and wash your hands.

PROCEDURE 16-5 *Rapid Strep Test*

To perform a rapid strep test for strep throat, you will need the following equipment and supplies:

- Directing Strep A test kit
- Throat swab specimen
- Wristwatch with a "sweep" second hand

Method

1. Gather all supplies and equipment needed to perform the test.
2. Wash hands and don gloves and face protection.
3. Position all bottles vertically and dispense reagents slowly as free-falling drops.
4. Add three drops of reagent 1 to an extraction tube. This solution is pink.

5. Add three drops of reagent 2 to the same tube. The solution should turn yellow.
6. Place the specimen swab in the tube, twirling the swab in the mix.
7. Wait for exactly 1 minute.
8. Add three drops of reagent 3 to the same tube, again twirling the swab in the tube to mix. This solution should be pink.
9. Discard the swab in a biohazard waste container.
10. Remove the reaction disk from the pouch and place it on a dry, flat surface.
11. Pour the entire contents of the tube into the reaction disk.
12. Read the test results when the entire end of the assay window turns red (5–10 minutes).
13. Dispose all contaminated waste.
14. Clean work area, remove gloves, and wash your hands.

Visit www.pearsonhighered.com/healthprofessionsresources to access figures and tables available on the student resources website. Click on view all resources and select Medical Assisting from the choice of disciplines. Find this book and you can see all respective tables and figures.

CHAPTER 17
Urinalysis

Urine is the most frequently analyzed body fluid other than blood. Accuracy of test results depends on the following:

- Collection methods
- Transportation and handling of specimens
- Types of containers used
- Timeliness of testing to prevent multiplication of bacteria and breakdown of components such as bilirubin and cellular elements.

COMPOSITION OF NORMAL URINE

It is important to understand the normal values of urine when conducting urinalysis. Table 17-1 gives normal urine values.

Collecting the Urine Specimen

Urine must be properly collected, and the method used is dependent upon the tests required to be performed on the specimen. The following are various methods of urine collection:

- Fasting specimen
- First morning specimen (first thing in morning after approximately 8 hours of sleep)
- Random specimen (collected at any time)
- Twenty-four-hour specimen
- Two-hour postprandial specimen

Table 17-1 *Normal Values for Urinalysis Testing*

Element	Normal Values
Appearance	Clear, slightly cloudy
Bilirubin	Negative
Blood	Negative
Color	Straw, pale yellow, yellow, darker yellow, amber
Glucose	Negative
Ketone	Negative
Leukocytes	Negative
Nitrites	Negative
Odor	Aromatic
Protein	Negative to trace
Reaction/pH	4.6–7.9
Specific gravity	1.010–1.030
Urobilinogen	Less than 2 Ehrlich units/dL

Specialized Collection

These collections include

- Catheterized specimen (sterile)
- Clean-catch midstream (sterile specimen)
- Suprapubic specimen (sterile specimen)
- Pediatric specimen

Labeling

The medical assistant must label all specimens. The following information is included on the label:

- Patient's first and last name

- Date and time of collection
- Patient's date of birth
- Initials of person performing the collection
- Timed specimen (collected at specific times)
  - Tolerance tests (glucose tolerance test) such as fasting, 1/2 hour, and 1 hour
  - Twenty-four-hour test (collected to allow quantitative analysis of urine analyte)

Collection of a 24-hour specimen requires a large, clean, and wide-mouthed container that can hold several liters.

Key Focus: A random urine sample is the most commonly collected type of urine specimen.

COMMON URINE TESTS

A routine urinalysis is the analysis of a urine specimen and includes

- Physical analysis
- Chemical analysis
- Microscopic examination

Physical Analysis

Physical analysis of urine characteristics includes

- Color—ranging from light straw to dark amber
- Odor
- Specific gravity (concentration)—methods include
  - Dipstick or reagent strip (most commonly used method)
  - Refractometer
  - Urinometer (less commonly used today)
- Quantity (volume)

Specific gravity may be high or low in various conditions or disorders (see Table 17-2).

> **Key Focus:** Specific gravity is the weight of a substance related to the same amount of distilled water; it indicates how the kidneys concentrate or dilute urine.

Chemical Characteristics

Chemical composition is most commonly determined by the use of a plastic strip containing areas impregnated with reagents (commonly called a "dipstick"). Reagent strips can be used to analyze the presence of the following:

- Bacteria
- Blood
- Bilirubin
- Urobilinogen
- Nitrite
- Glucose
- Ketones

Table 17-2 *Abnormal Specific Gravity*

High	Low
Adrenal cortex deficiency	Chronic renal disorders
Diabetes mellitus	Diabetes insipidus
Dehydration	Excessive hydration
Heart failure	Glomerulonephritis
Hepatic disease	Pyelonephritis

- Leukocytes
- pH
- Protein
- Specific gravity

Microscopic Examination

Microscopic examination identifies the type and approximate numbers of organisms present in a urine specimen. When examined under a microscope, urine components such as cells, crystals, and microorganisms can be seen. Table 17-3 lists routine urinalysis categories.

Table 17-3 *Routine Urinalysis Categories*

Physical	Chemical	Microscopic
	Bilirubin	
	Blood	
	Glucose	
	Ketones	Blood (RBCs, WBCs)
Appearance (clarity or turbidity)	Leukocytes	Casts (hyaline, cellular, granular, waxy)
Color	Nitrite	Cells
Odor	Protein	Crystals (acid/lkaline)
Quantity (24-hour specimen only)	Reaction (pH)	Epithelial cells
Specific gravity	Urobilinogen	Others: bacteria, spermatozoa, parasites, yeast

Urinalysis

GUIDELINES FOR COLLECTING A ROUTINE URINE SAMPLE

The following steps are required to collect a routine urine sample:

- Provide the patient with a nonsterile container labeled with the patient's name and the date of collection.
- Ask the patient to use the bathroom and void into the container.
- Tell the patient only to fill the container 2/3 of the way to avoid spillage.
- Explain where you want the patient to leave the container.
- Place a waterproof pad in the designated area to avoid contamination of the work area.
- Wear nonsterile gloves during the procedure.
- Test the urine immediately if possible.
- If unable to test the urine within 30 minutes, place it in a refrigerator. The urine, however, should be allowed to warm up to room temperature before testing.

PROCEDURE 17-1 *Collecting a Clean-Catch Specimen*

Both male and female patients must correctly provide a contaminant-free, clean-catch midstream urine specimen using the following equipment and supplies:

- Antiseptic towelettes
- Sterile urine container
- Written patient instructions

Method

1. Perform hand hygiene.
2. Assemble equipment.

3. Identify and greet the patient.
4. Explain the procedure to a female patient as follows:
   - Wash hands, remove underwear.
   - Expose urinary meatus by pulling apart labia, holding open with nondominant hand.
   - Use the dominant hand to cleanse around the area.
   - Begin voiding into the toilet.
   - Place the container into position and void into it without touching the inside of the container with the fingers.
   - Remove the container and continue voiding into the toilet.
   - Wipe in the usual manner and cover the container with its lid.
   - Avoid contaminating the inside of the lid by not touching it.
   - Deliver the specimen as instructed.
5. Explain the procedure to a male patient as follows:
   - Wash hands and expose the penis.
   - Pull the foreskin back (if uncircumcised) and hold back until the specimen has been collected.
   - Cleanse each side of the urethral opening from the top to the bottom, wiping in one direction only.
   - Void a small amount of urine into the toilet, then void into the container.
   - Do not touch the inside of the container.
   - Remove the container.
   - Continue voiding the remainder of urine into the toilet.
   - Recap the container being careful not to touch the inside of the lid.
   - Deliver the specimen as instructed.
6. Label the specimen container.
7. Document the chart appropriately.

Urinalysis

PROCEDURE 17-2 *Physical Urinalysis*

Urinalysis begins with the physical examination and the evaluation of the physical characteristics of urine using the following equipment and supplies:

- Urine specimen
- Centrifuge tube
- Laboratory slip
- Personal protective equipment (as needed)

Method

1. Perform hand hygiene and wear gloves.
2. Mix the urine by carefully swirling it.
3. Label the centrifuge tube with the patient's name.
4. Assess the color of the specimen and record it.
5. Assess the odor of the specimen and record it.
6. Assess the clarity and record it using appropriate terms (clear, slightly cloudy, cloudy, or turbid).
7. Clean the area.
8. Remove the gloves.

PROCEDURE 17-3 *Measuring Specific Gravity*

Measuring specific gravity with a refractometer should be performed without error and is conducted using the following equipment and supplies:

- Refractometer
- Paper towels
- Pipettes
- Medicine droppers
- Protective eyewear
- Laboratory coat
- Gloves

- Urine specimen
- Distilled water

Method

1. Perform hand hygiene.
2. Wear gloves and protective clothing.
3. Assemble the equipment and materials.
4. Perform a quality control check by using a sample of distilled water—the value should be 1.000.
5. Place one to two drops of urine onto the notched area of the cover.
6. Read the specific gravity.
7. Record the reading on a piece of paper.
8. Discard the urine appropriately.
9. Remove gloves and perform hand hygiene.
10. Document the findings in the patient record.
11. Clean the work area and equipment.

Key Focus: The presence of glucose, protein, or x-ray dyes may increase the specific gravity of urine.

PROCEDURE 17-4 *Testing Urine with Reagent Strips*

Chemical testing of urine using chemical strips (dipsticks) is very common in the medical office and uses the following equipment and supplies:

- Urine specimen
- Reagent test strips
- Timer
- Paper towels

- Laboratory slip
- Personal protective equipment as needed

Method

1. Perform hand hygiene and put on personal protective equipment.
2. Check the specimen for patient identity, date, and time of collection.
3. Check the expiration date on the chemical reagent strips.
4. Dip a chemical reagent strip in urine, making sure that all pads on the strip are moistened (see Figure 17-1A).

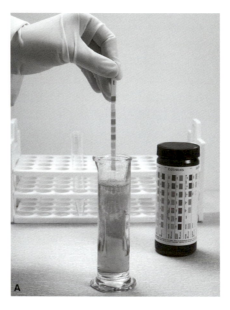

Figure 17-1 *(A) Dip reagent strip into urine; (Continued)*

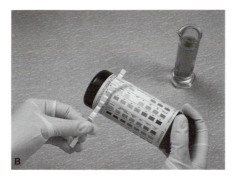

Figure 17-1 *(B) compare strip to chart. (Continued)*

5. Always be sure to hold the strip horizontally when reading.
6. Read each pad by comparing it to the chart on the side of the bottle appropriately timing each test.
7. Record the results on the patient's laboratory slip.
8. Clean the work area, remove gloves, and complete the patient's chart.

MICROSCOPIC URINE SAMPLE

Microscopic examination of urine sediment for casts and cells is the last step of urinalysis and uses the following equipment and supplies:

- Personal protective equipment as needed (laboratory coat, nonsterile gloves)
- Capillary pipettes
- Centrifuge
- Centrifuge tubes
- Microscope

- Microscope slides
- Urine specimen

> **Key Focus:** Microscopic examination of urine is out of the scope of practice of the medical assistant.

PROCEDURE 17-5 *Urine Pregnancy Testing*

This type of pregnancy testing is based on the detection of human chorionic gonadotropin (hCG), which is produced by the placenta and is present in the urine of pregnant women.

The following equipment and supplies are used:

- An early morning urine specimen
- Enzyme immunoassay (EIA) test kit for hCG
- Gloves
- Timer
- Laboratory report

Method

1. Perform hand hygiene and wear gloves.
2. Assemble equipment and supplies.
3. Label the test with the patient's name or ID number.
4. Label one area positive and one area negative (for control).
5. Place the patient's urine on the test chamber following the manufacturer's directions.
6. Place positive and negative controls in the correct areas.
7. Time the test according to the manufacturer's directions.
8. Interpret the results correctly.
9. Record the results.
10. Dispose of the equipment and perform hand hygiene.

CHAPTER 18
Medical Emergencies

In all emergencies involving injuries or illnesses, follow these basic steps:

- Recognize emergency, check scene
- Decide to help
- Check the patient
- Call 911 (when appropriate)
- Give first aid
- Seek medical attention

BASIC LIFE SUPPORT

Basic life support (BLS) refers to first aid given if patient's breathing or heart stops—often needed for patients of

- Heart attack
- Drowning
- Choking

Cardiac Arrest

Cardiac arrest refers to the heartbeat suddenly stopping. Causes of sudden cardiac arrest include

- Heart attack
- Certain heart medications
- Drug abuse or overdose
- Electrocution
- Drowning
- Choking
- Traumatic injury

CPR FOR ADULTS

"A-B-C-D's" of cardiopulmonary resuscitation (CPR):

- Airway
- Breathing
- Circulation
- Defibrillation

CPR Protocol

- Shake and shout.
- Call for help; call 911.
- Check for back/neck injury.
- Open airway; check for breathing.
- Clear foreign bodies (if necessary).
- Ventilate the patient with two effective breaths.
- Check carotid pulse for 5–10 seconds.
- Initiate CPR at 30 cardiac compressions to two ventilations, at a rate of 100 compressions per minute.
- Check for carotid pulse after 1 minute; if absent, continue CPR.

PROCEDURE 18-1 *Steps of CPR*

1. Feel for carotid pulse; palpate one side with two fingers for 5–10 seconds (Figure 18-1).
2. Check for other signs of circulation (normal breathing, coughing, movement in response to rescue breaths).
3. If pulse or other signs of circulation are not present, begin CPR.
   - Position yourself next to the patient, on their left side, near their head.
   - Position your hands on the lower half of the sternum right between the nipples.

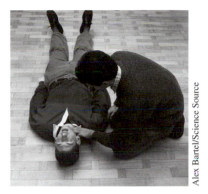

Alex Bartel/Science Source

Figure 18-1 *Feel for pulse.*

- Place heel of one hand on the sternum and other hand superimposed on top of the first hand.
- Interlace the fingers and extend the fingers off the rib cage (Figure 18-2).

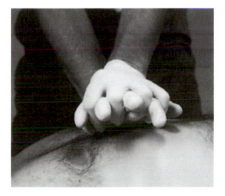

Figure 18-2 *Position hands.*

- If trained in CPR, administer 30 compressions at a rate of 100 compressions per minute; compress chest 1½–2 inches. If not trained, administer uninterrupted compressions without rescue breathing.
- Count compressions.
- Release pressure between compressions for cardiac refilling; do not take heel of hand off chest.
4. Continue CPR in a cycle of 30 compressions and two rescue breaths for a single rescuer.
5. Pause 2 seconds for each ventilation.
6. Check carotid pulse for 5 seconds after four cycles of compression and ventilation.

PROCEDURE 18-2 *CPR for Airway*

1. Press backward on forehead for opening the airway.
2. Place two fingers on the chin and lift it up.
3. Evaluate respiratory function.
   - Put your ear down near the patient's mouth and nose.
   - Look for chest movement.
   - Feel for airflow against your cheek.
   - Listen for exhalation of breath.

PROCEDURE 18-3 *CPR for Rescue Breathing*

1. Evaluate respiratory function.
   - Put your ear down near the patient's mouth and nose.
   - Look for chest movement.
   - Feel for airflow against your cheek.
   - Listen for exhalation of breath.
2. Prepare to ventilate if no respiration is present.
   - Leave dentures in place.
   - Pinch off nostrils.

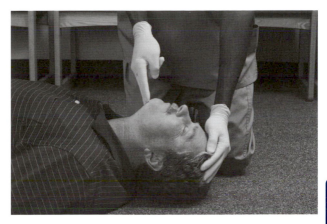

Figure 18-3 *A medical assistant performs a head tilt.*

- Fully cover the patient's mouth to form a mouth-to-mouth seal, or place barrier device on patient's face and place your mouth on breathing piece or opening.
- Continue to tilt the head and lift the chin before each ventilation.
- Tilt head back to maintain open airway (see Figure 18-3).
- Monitor patient closely until transported to a medical facility.

Key Focus: The earlier defibrillation occurs, the better chance of survival. When ventricular fibrillation is present, CPR can provide small amounts of blood to heart and brain.

AED Operation

Use automated external defibrillators (AEDs) only when patients have the following three clinical findings:

- No response
- No breathing
- No pulse

PROCEDURE 18-4 *Using an AED*

The common steps to operate all AEDs include

- Open the AED and press the power button on.
- Place the AED near the head on the left side of patient.
- Remove patient's clothing on his or her torso.
- If the patient has a medicine patch in the same place where you would attach the AED patch, take the medicine patch off (while wearing gloves).
- Quickly wipe the chest where the medicine patch was before you put on the AED patch.
- Ensure chest is dry (also, if the patient is in a wet environment, they should be moved to a drier place).
- If the patient has a hairy chest, apply AED patches and then remove them quickly to remove the patient's hair.
- Open package of new adhesive electrode patches.
- Peel off protective plastic backing from patches to expose adhesive surface.
- Place two patches directly on the skin of the chest using the following steps:
  - First patch goes on the upper right side of the patient's chest, to the right of the sternum, with the top edge touching the bottom of the clavicle.
  - Second patch (marked with a ♥) goes to outside of the left nipple, with top margin of patch at anterior axillary line.

- Do not place patches directly over nitroglycerin patches or within 5 inches of implanted devices such as pacemakers.
- Stop CPR if CPR is being performed.
- Turn the AED on and connect leads to the patches.
- Instruct everyone helping not to touch the patient in order to analyze rhythm.
- Push ANALYZE button to start the analysis. Some machines begin analyzing rhythm as soon as patches are applied.
- If analysis indicates need for a shock, push SHOCK on the AED. A voice message will inform everyone to "stay clear." A good way to make sure that no one is touching the patient prior to shock is the "I'm clear, you're clear, we're all clear" procedure.
- Press ANALYZE button if necessary.
- If patient is not in need of shock, rescuer should immediately check for pulse and begin CPR.

Key Focus: If you are using a fully automated AED, you may not have to press a button for the AED to analyze or shock the patient.

Outcome and Actions After Shock Delivery

Follow these steps after the AED delivers a shock to the patient:

- Immediately resume CPR beginning with chest compressions.
- After five cycles (about 2 minutes) of CPR, allow the AED to analyze the heart rhythm. If a shock is not advised, resume CPR for five more cycles.
- Continue until advanced care providers take over, or the patient starts to move.

Special Situations Using an AED

The following five special situations may require the operator to take additional actions when using an AED:

- The patient is less than 1 year of age.
- The patient has a hairy chest.
- The patient is immersed in water or water is covering their chest.
- The patient has an implanted defibrillator or pacemaker.
- The patient has a transdermal medication patch or other object on surface of skin where the AED electrode pads are placed.

> **Key Focus:** Currently, there is not enough evidence to recommend for or against the use of AEDs in infants less than 1 year of age.

CPR FOR CHILDREN

Medical assistants should use child CPR guidelines for children from 1 year of age to puberty. Once a child reaches puberty, you should use adult CPR guidelines for resuscitation.

Modifications to CPR for Children

Although the steps for giving CPR to an adult and a child are similar, there are a few differences:

- Amount of air for breaths
- Possible need to try more than twice to deliver two breaths that make the chest rise
- Depth of compressions
- May use one-handed chest compressions for very small children
- What to do when the child's pulse is less than 60 beats per minute

- When to attach an AED
- When to activate the emergency response system

PROCEDURE 18-5 *Administering CPR to Children*

The following steps should be taken for giving CPR to a child:

- Assess the patient for a response; if no response, shout for help.
- If someone responds, send that person to activate the emergency response system and get an AED (if available).
- Open the patient's airway and assess their breathing (take at least 5 seconds but no more than 10 seconds).
- If not breathing, give two breaths.
- Check the patient's pulse (take between 5 and 10 seconds). If there is no pulse, or if the heart rate is less than 60 beats per minute, perform cycles of compressions and ventilations (30:2 ratio) at a rate of 100 compressions per minute.
- After five cycles of CPR
  - If someone has not done this, activate the emergency response system and get an AED, if available.
  - Use the AED; for children, this requires an adaptor to lower the voltage.

CPR for Infants

The term *infant* includes the neonatal period outside the delivery room setting and extends to 1 year of age (12 months). The infant BLS sequence includes

- Airway
- Breathing
- Circulation

Medical Emergencies

Chest Compression Technique

Chest compressions to an infant follow these steps:

- Place the infant on a firm, flat surface.
- Remove clothing from the infant's chest.
- Draw an imaginary line between the nipples.
- Place two fingers on the breastbone just below this line.
- Press the infant's breastbone down about 1/3 to 1/2 of the depth of the chest.
- After each compression, completely release the pressure on the breastbone and allow the chest to recoil completely.
- Deliver compressions at a rate of 100 compressions per minute.

Table 18-1 outlines the basic differences in rates and ratios between adult, child, and infant CPR.

HEIMLICH MANEUVER FOR CHOKING

Choking occurs when food or a foreign object blocks an individual's trachea. The patient is usually not able to speak. Figure 18-4 displays the Heimlich maneuver. The following is the procedure to use:

- Ask "Are you choking?"
- Ask "Can you speak?"
- Tell the patient you are going to help them.
- Walk around behind the patient.
- Encircle the patient with your arms.
- Locate the navel and the bottom end of the sternum (the xiphoid process).
- Place the thumb side of your closed fist against the patient's abdomen directly between these two points.
- Grab your fist with your other hand and deliver a firm thrust into the patient's abdomen in an upward direction toward you.

Table 18-1 *Adult Versus Pediatric CPR Rates and Ratios*

Healthcare Provider Technique	Adult	Child	Infant
Compressions/breaths	30:2	30:2	30:2
Compressions/minute	100	100	100
Compression	1½–2 inches	1/3–1/2 the depth of the child's chest (approximately)	1/3–1/2 the depth of the infant's chest (approximately)
Breaths/minute	10–12	12–20	12–20
Breaths, duration in seconds	1 (one breath every 5–6 seconds)	1 (one breath every 3–5 seconds)	1 (one breath every 3–5 seconds)
Hand(s) on sternum	Two hands/lower half	One hand/lower half	Two fingers/lower third

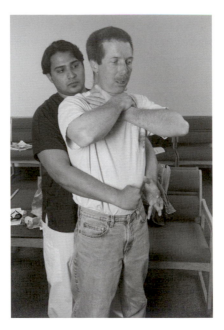

Figure 18-4 *Heimlich maneuver.*

- Keep doing that until the patient coughs up the obstruction or until they lose consciousness.

BURNS

A burn injury occurs when an area of tissue is destroyed by the action of

- Physical heat
- Chemical activity
- High electrical current
- Heavy exposure to radon

Table 18-2 *Classification of Burns*

Degree	Characteristics
First	Reddening, swelling of the epidermis (similar to a mild sunburn)
Second	Reddening, swelling of the epidermis and outer dermis; blistering
Third	Charring of all layers of skin and at least some deeper structures

Burns are classified by surface area and depth. Table 18-2 shows the classifications of burns.

Rule of Nines

The Rule of Nines is a useful tool for calculating the percentage of body surface affected by burns in adults, children, and infants (except for the genital region). See Figure 18-5.

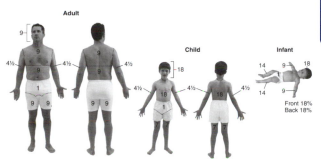

Note: Each arm totals 9% (front of arm 4½%, back of arm 4½%)

Figure 18-5 *Rule of Nines.*

BONE FRACTURES

A bone fracture is a break or crack in a bone. Table 18-3 lists various types of fractures. Figure 18-6 shows some examples of fractures.

Table 18-3 *Types of Bone Fractures*

Fracture	Description
Closed (simple)	Ends of fractured bone do not break through skin
Open (compound)	Ends of fractured bone break through skin
Complete	Bone is completely broken into two or more pieces
Incomplete	Bone is partially broken
Greenstick	Bone is bent on one side and has an incomplete fracture on the opposite side
Hairline	Bone has fine cracks but bone sections remain in place
Comminuted	Bone is broken into three or more pieces
Displaced	Ends of fractured bone move out of the normal position
Nondisplaced	Ends of fractured bone stay in the normal position
Impacted	Piece of broken bone is forced into a space of another bone fragment
Depressed	Fractured bone forms a concavity; mostly seen in skull fractures

Table 18-3 (*Continued*)

Fracture	Description
Linear	Fracture is parallel to the long axis of the bone
Transverse	Fracture is perpendicular to the long axis of the bone
Oblique	Fracture runs diagonally across the bone
Spiral	Fracture spirals around long axis of bone, usually the result of twisting a bone
Colles	Fracture is at the distal end of the radius or ulna
Pott	Fracture is at the distal end of tibia or fibula

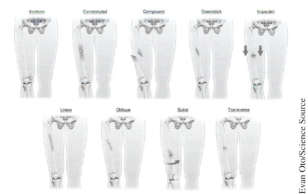

Evan Oto/Science Source

Figure 18-6 *Fractures.*

BONE-RELATED INJURIES

- Dislocation—separation of two bones where they meet at a joint; they are no longer in normal positions
- Sprain—a stretched or torn ligament, which is the tissue that connects bones at a joint
- Strain—a stretched or torn muscle or tendon; a tendon is the tissue that connects muscles to bones

HEAD INJURIES

- Concussion—a common, jarring brain injury; patient may lose consciousness and vision temporarily
  - Other symptoms include paleness, listlessness, memory loss, and vomiting lasting up to 24 hours
  - May potentially cause slow intracranial bleeding— teach patients and families what to do
- Contusion—a severe injury involving bruising
- Hematoma—swelling caused by blood under the skin; can be reduced by applying ice immediately
- Laceration—when occurring in the scalp, profuse bleeding may occur that is less serious than it appears
  - Apply direct pressure to stop bleeding
  - Wash area with soap and water
  - Apply a dry, sterile dressing
- Other severe head injuries include fractures and intracranial bleeding—immediate hospitalization required
  - M.A. must monitor circulation, airway, breathing; begin CPR if needed

HEMORRHAGING

It is heavy or uncontrollable bleeding, usually from injury but also from illness—can be internal or external.

- If internal bleeding is suspected, cover the patient with a blanket, encourage quiet and calmness, and seek immediate medical help.
- Control external bleeding to prevent rapid blood loss and shock.
  - Use direct pressure, apply additional dressings if needed.
  - Elevate the bleeding body part, and put pressure over a pressure point.
  - Transport patient to an emergency care facility.
- If medical help is more than an hour away, a tourniquet may be needed.
  - Apply tourniquet over the main pressure point above the wound.
  - Tighten tourniquet until bleeding stops.
  - For upper limbs, place tourniquet as high as possible, tighten as much as possible.
  - Write tourniquet's application time on tourniquet or on patient's forehead.
  - Proper use of tourniquets may stop life-threatening hemorrhage without loss of affected limb.

WEATHER-RELATED INJURIES

- Heatstroke—overheating due to prolonged exposure to high temperature and humidity; may lead to excessive dehydration and hypovolemic shock
  - Temperature over 104°F can damage tissues and organs, leading to death
  - Symptoms: hot and dry skin, altered mental state, rapid pulse and breathing, dizziness, headache, nausea and vomiting, weakness, and high body temperature
  - Check CAB's and call EMS system; move patient to a cool place and remove outer clothing if needed

- Cool patient with gentle spraying of water, fan the patient, or apply a wet sheet
- If humidity is above 75%, place ice packs on patient's groin and armpits
- Stop cooling when patient's mental state improves
- Keep patient's head and shoulders slightly elevated
- Sunburn—redness, tenderness, pain, swelling, blisters, and peeling skin; can lead to skin damage or cancer
  - Soak skin in cool water; apply cold compresses, and later, calamine lotion
  - Have patient elevate legs and arms to prevent swelling
  - Have patient drink plenty of water and take a pain reliever
  - Patients must be educated about applying sunscreen every 2–3 hours when outdoors, and stay out of direct sunlight between 10:00 a.m. and 2:00 p.m., which is when rays are strongest
- Hypothermia—occurs when body temperature drops below 95°F, due to exposure to the cold
  - Symptoms: lethargy, loss of coordination, confusion, and uncontrollable shivering
  - If untreated, it can result in cardiac arrest and coma
  - Move patient inside if possible, and cover with blankets; remove wet clothing
  - If patient is confused or unconscious, monitor breathing and call EMS system
  - If patient is awake and alert, give warm liquids that do not contain alcohol
- Frostbite—occurs when tissues are exposed to temperatures lower than freezing; ice crystals form between tissue cells, and enlarge as they extract cellular water; may lead to blood clots and severe cellular damage

- Symptoms: white, waxy, or grayish yellow skin; affected area feels cold, tingling, and painful; skin feels crusty
- If frostbite is deep, body part may feel cold and hard and not be sensitive to pain
- Blisters may appear after rewarming; do not break blisters
- Wrap warm clothing or blankets around body part, or place it in contact with a warm body part
- If in a remote area, use the wet rapid rewarming method: place affected part in 100°F to 104°F water; add hot water regularly to keep temperature stable; alternative method is to use warm compresses for 20–40 minutes
- Do not rub or massage the affected area—this can further damage tissues
- If affected area becomes soft, place dry sterile gauze between skin surfaces

POISONING

It is extremely important that the medical assistant calls a poison-control center, hospital emergency department, doctor, or the emergency medical service (EMS) system for instructions. You will need to know the following:

- The patient's name and age
- The name of the poison
- The amount of poison swallowed
- Whether the poison was ingested, absorbed, or inhaled
- When the poison was swallowed
- Whether or not the person has vomited
- How much time it will take to get the patient to a medical facility
- The National Hotline for Poison Control is 1-800-222-1222

BITES AND STINGS

The most common bites involve dogs and cats, with less common bites involving snakes and spiders. The most common stings involve bees, wasps, and hornets.

Animal Bites

An animal bite that breaks the skin should be treated by a physician, and must be reported to the police, animal control, and local health department.

- If the animal is found, it must be checked for rabies; it may need to be quarantined
- If the animal is not found, patient may receive precautionary rabies immunoglobulins and vaccination
- The animals most commonly carrying rabies are dogs, cats, skunks, squirrels, raccoons, bats, and foxes
- Bites from other humans may transmit HIV or hepatitis B; for hep-B, series of three immunizations are given
- For any bite, wash the area with antiseptic soap and water; apply a dry sterile dressing
  - If bleeding profusely or spurting blood, apply pressure and seek medical attention
  - Tetanus toxoid should be administered if the patient has not received it in 5–10 years

SNAKEBITES

The most common poisonous snakes in the United States include rattlesnakes, water moccasins (cottonmouths), copperheads, coral snakes. Bites produce two puncture marks, pain, swelling at the site, rarely leading to death.

- Additional symptoms: rapid pulse, nausea, vomiting, and sometimes unconsciousness and seizures.
- If possible, describe the snake to EMS or the hospital so that correct antivenin can be administered.

- If a potentially poisoning snakebite occurs, call a physician or the EMS system.
- Walking should be avoided, but if the patient must walk, do it slowly to avoid spreading the poison.
  - Keep patient calm, and remove rings, watches, or tight clothing near the bite.
  - Immobilize the injured part, and position it below heart level.
  - Do not apply ice or a tourniquet; do not cut or suction the wound.

SPIDER BITES

Two types of poisonous spiders in the United States are as follows:

- Black widow—red hourglass mark on its abdomen; bite causes swelling and pain at site, then nausea, vomiting, rigid abdomen, fever, rash, and difficulty breathing or swallowing
- Brown recluse—violin-shaped mark on its head; bite causes severe swelling, tenderness, and then ulceration around the bite location

Any patient bitten by a spider requires medical attention.

- Wash bite with soap and water, apply a cold compress to reduce swelling and pain; elevate the area
- Healing can sometimes take several months

INSECT STINGS

Insect stings may become red, swollen, itchy, and painful. For a honeybee sting, the stinger must be removed to stop it from continually releasing venom—scrape the skin with a flat and sharp object. Do not use your fingers or tweezers to try and remove the stinger, otherwise more venom may be released.

- If a honeybee stinger cannot be removed, call a physician. Wash with soap and water.
- If the stinger is removed, apply ice for 10 minutes with 10-minute breaks as needed for pain and swelling.
- An insect sting can be deadly, causing anaphylaxis, if the patient is allergic to venom.

SECTION V

Basic Pharmacology and Administration of Medications

Basic
Pharmacology

CHAPTER 19
Principles of Pharmacology

Pharmacology is a dynamic science involving the study of how drugs affect living organisms and the uses of drugs. Medical assistants must understand

- Drug actions
- Adverse effects
- Routes of administration
- Recommended doses
- Effects of drugs on individual patients
- Drug interactions
- Drug absorption
- Drug distribution
- Drug metabolism
- Drug elimination

PHARMACOKINETICS

Pharmacokinetics is the pharmaceutical science studying the time it takes for a drug to be effective. It involves the movement of a drug in the body. Pharmacokinetics consists of four steps:

1. Absorption (through the GI tract, by injection, or other routes of administration, such as transdermal applications, inhalation, nasal, ophthalmic, otic, vaginal, and rectal)
2. Metabolism (occurs in the liver)
3. Distribution (through the blood circulation)
4. Excretion (elimination from the body)

PHARMACODYNAMICS

Pharmacodynamics is the study of the interaction of drugs with their sites of action. It examines the way drugs bind with their receptors and the concentration required to elicit a response. Pharmacodynamics focuses on

- Mechanism of action
- Drug interactions

DRUG NAMES

- Generic name (official name)
- Trade names (brand or proprietary names)—selected by manufacturers and protected by copyright
- Chemical name (international nonproprietary name)

Prescriptions and Interpreting

Drugs not available over the counter require prescriptions. Medical assistants must interpret prescriptions to discuss them with patients, prescribers, and pharmacists. The basic components of prescriptions include

- Prescriber information—name, address, phone number, other identifying information
- Patient information—full name, date of birth, address, other identifying information
- Medication prescribed—generic or brand name, strength, quantity (called *inscription*, found after the *Rx*)
- Subscription—instructions to pharmacist, including generic substitution and refill authorization
- Signa (transcription)—patient instructions (usually follow abbreviation *Sig*, which means "mark")
- Prescriber's signature—for handwritten prescriptions, must be in ink and cannot be stamped
  - Digital signature used if secure—otherwise, prescription is printed, signed, or authorized

- Prescriber must include the date the prescription was written
- DEA number—required for Schedule II, III, IV, and V medications

Abbreviations should be avoided for drug names. Also, the "Do Not Use" list of abbreviations should be followed.

E-Prescriptions

E-prescribing is the entering of information electronically, for direct transmission. This avoids having the patient receiving a written prescription, and is the most secure, efficient method of prescribing.

- Provides automatic drug and allergy interaction checking
- Eliminates medication errors due to poor handwriting
- Greatly reduces communications from pharmacies requesting prescription clarifications
- The national clearinghouse for e-prescribing is called "Surescripts"—providers can access prescription information to see patients' total history from all sources

Telephone Prescriptions

Medical assistants may be requested to phone in new or renewal prescriptions to pharmacies—except for Schedule II drugs (except in emergencies, wherein physicians can phone in for these prescriptions, then follow up with a written prescription within 72 hours).

GOVERNMENT REGULATION

The Food and Drug Administration (FDA), a division of the Department of Health and Human Services, regulates the development and sale of all prescription and over-the-counter (OTC) drugs.

Key Focus: The Drug Enforcement Administration (DEA) is the law enforcement agency responsible for the control of narcotics and drug abuse, the illegal sale of dangerous substances, and drug abuse prevention through public education.

Controlled Substances

Based on guidelines set forth by Controlled Substances Act (CSA), controlled substances are divided into five schedules (see Table 19-1).

Table 19-1 *Schedules of Controlled Substances*

Schedule	Description	Examples
I	High potential for abuse; no medical use in the United States; lack of accepted safety	Cannabis (except for approved use),* heroin, LSD, peyote, mescaline, etc.
II	High potential for abuse; currently accepted medical use with restrictions in the United States; abuse may lead to severe physical or psychological dependence	Cocaine, methylphenidate, phenylcyclohexyl piperidine, opium, oxycodone, morphine, secobarbital, methamphetamine, etc.
III	Less abuse potential than Schedules I and II; currently	Anabolic steroids, talbutal, paregoric, Marinol,

Schedule	Description	Examples
	accepted medical use in the United States; abuse may lead to moderate or low physical dependence, or high psychological dependence	hydrocodone/ codeine, etc.
IV	Low abuse potential; currently accepted medical use in the United States; abuse may lead to limited physical or psychological dependence	Diazepam, zolpidem, phenobarbital, pentazocine, pemoline, etc.
V	Low abuse potential; currently accepted medical use in the United States; abuse may lead to limited physical or psychological dependence; most Schedule V drugs are available without a prescription	Cough suppressants containing small amounts of codeine, preparations containing small amounts of opium or diphenoxylate, pregabalin, etc.

*There is controversy about the placement of cannabis in Schedule I because it now has some approved medical uses in certain countries and many U.S. states.

Important Guidelines for Handling Controlled Substances

- Any drug loss must be reported to regional DEA office or local law enforcement immediately.
- If a controlled substance is damaged, outdated, or must be disposed of (e.g., a pill falls onto the floor during dispensing), two employees must be present to witness its proper disposal according to new government guidelines; both must document procedure on the controlled substances inventory form used by the office.
- The government now recommends the following procedures for proper drug disposal:
  - Take unused, unneeded, or expired prescription drugs out of their original containers.
  - Mix them with an undesirable substance such as coffee grounds or cat litter.
  - Put the mixture in an empty can or sealable bag, and throw in the trash.
  - When possible, return prescription drugs to pharmaceutical take-back locations.
  - Drugs prone to diversion still should be flushed, including
    - Actiq (fentanyl citrate)
    - Daytrana transdermal patch (methylphenidate)
    - Duragesic transdermal system (fentanyl)
    - OxyContin tablets (oxycodone)
    - Avinza capsules (morphine sulfate)
    - Baraclude tablets (entecavir)
    - Reyataz capsules (atazanavir sulfate)
    - Tequin tablets (gatifloxacin)
    - Zerit for oral solution (stavudine)
    - Meperidine HCl tablets
    - Percocet (oxycodone/acetaminophen)

- Xyrem (sodium oxybate)
  - Fentora (fentanyl buccal tablet)
- If a large quantity of scheduled drugs must be disposed of, contact local DEA office for guidance.

Prescription Guidelines for Controlled Substances

The following guidelines must be followed when writing prescriptions:

- The prescription must be written in ink or typed using a computer or typewriter.
- It must include the following:
  - Patient's name and address
  - Physician's name, address, and DEA number
  - Date the medication was prescribed
- The amount prescribed must be written out (e.g., "five" rather than "5").
- The prescription must be manually signed by the physician.
- Drugs in Schedules II, III, and IV must include the following statement on their label: Federal law prohibits the transfer of this drug to any person other than the patient for whom it is ordered.

Specific Rules

The symbols C-II, C-III, C-IV, and C-V are used to indicate drugs from each schedule. Prescription guidelines for each schedule are located in Table 19-2.

Common Controlled Substances

- Anabolic steroids
- Butabarbital

Table 19-2 *Drug Schedules and Prescription Guidelines*

Schedule	Prescription Guideline
II (C-II)	These prescriptions must be written (unless an absolute emergency exists that requires a telephone order for the prescription) These prescriptions cannot be refilled Certain states require the use of multiple-copy prescriptions to ensure that proper documentation of these prescriptions is made and retained
III (C-III)	These prescriptions may be oral or written Within 6 months of original prescription, prescriptions may be refilled (up to five times)
IV (C-IV)	These prescriptions may be oral, written, or electronic These prescriptions may be refilled up to five times
V (C-V)	These prescriptions may be oral, written, or electronic These prescriptions may be refilled up to five times Pharmacists may dispense these drugs without a prescription in certain states

- Chloral hydrate
- Cocaine
- Codeine
- Diazepam
- Heroin

- Lysergic acid diethylamide (LSD)
- Marijuana
- Morphine
- Opium
- Phenobarbital
- Secobarbital
- Tylenol with codeine

DRUG ABUSE

Drug abuse is defined as the use of a drug improperly or wrongly. Medical assistants must be aware of the potential for drug abuse and drug dependency in patients. Table 19-3 shows frequently abused drugs.

Key Focus: Medical assistants in most offices are responsible for an inventory of medications that are in stock, including samples from pharmaceutical companies.

DRUG CLASSIFICATIONS

Drug classifications are generally based on their actions. Table 19-4 shows drug classifications with names and

Table 19-3 *The Most Commonly Abused Drugs*

Sedatives	Anti-anxiety Drugs	Anti-depressants	Pain Medications	Illegal Drugs
Dalmane	Valium	Prozac	Demerol	Heroin
Restoril	Xanax	Elavil	Vicodin	Marijuana
Seconal	Librium	Tofranil	Percocet	Cocaine

descriptions of use. Table 19-5 presents classifications of drug types. These tables appear on the student resources website.

PHYSICIAN REGISTRATION

Authorized prescribers working with controlled substances must register with the DEA, have a current state medical license, and, sometimes, have a state controlled substance license.

- Registration, renewal, ordering of controlled substances must follow the Controlled Substances Act
- This includes registration, renewal, and ordering of controlled substances
- DEA Form 224 is used to register a practitioner

Drug Ordering

- DEA Form 222: to order scheduled drugs
- DEA Form 41: to dispose of scheduled drugs

Drug Security

- Controlled substances must be kept in locked cabinet or safe; double locks often used for opioids
- Licensed practitioners should keep the keys except when a medical assistant is allowed access
- If controlled drugs are stolen, call regional DEA office immediately; notify state bureau of narcotic enforcement and the local police
- File all reports required by the DEA and other agencies

Recordkeeping

Licensed practitioners who write prescriptions for controlled substances, as well as dispensing or administering them, must maintain two types of records:

- Inventory records of all stock on hand—applies to all scheduled drugs; inventory must occur every 2 years; must include copies of drug supplier invoices, with Schedule II drug information kept separate
- Dispensing records—kept separate from the patient's regular medical record; for every administration or dispensation, the practitioner must note the date, patient name and address, drug, quantity dispensed

Both types of records must be kept for 2 years, and may be inspected by the DEA. These two types of records are not needed if the physician only *writes* controlled drug prescriptions, and does not dispense or administer them.

Disposing of Drugs

Usually, biohazardous waste disposal companies handle disposal of outdated, noncontrolled drugs. According to the DEA, medications should never be flushed. They also should not be placed in the trash. For disposal of controlled drugs, including samples, DEA Form 41 must be used.

- Four copies of the form are completed, with the physician signing it
- The DEA should be called so that disposal instructions can be obtained; they will issue a receipt to the licensed practitioner, which must be kept secure

Any licensed practitioner who closes a practice must return DEA registration certificates and unused copies of DEA Form 222 to the nearest DEA office. The word "VOID" must be written across the fronts of these forms. Any remaining controlled drugs must be disposed of according to DEA regional office instructions.

DRUG INFORMATION SOURCES

The following sources should usually be available for easy access:

- The Physicians' Desk Reference (PDR)
- United States Pharmacopeia/National Formulary (USP/NF)
  - Published about every 5 years
  - Every drug listed must meet the strict guidelines of the USP/NF
- Drug evaluations
  - The American Medical Association (AMA) publishes annual drug evaluations
  - These drug evaluations contain information on more than 1,000 drugs (including their names, efficacy, adverse reactions, and precautions)
- American Hospital Formulary Service
  - Published by the American Society of Hospital Pharmacists
  - Generic drugs are listed based on drug actions

The Physicians' Desk Reference

The annual PDR has color-coded directories, as follows:

- Drug classifications
- Generic names
- Trade names
- Pharmaceutical company names
- Pharmaceutical company addresses
- Pharmaceutical company emergency contact information
- Pharmaceutical company telephone numbers
- Available drug products of each major pharmaceutical company

The drug information section of PDR is divided according to manufacturer subsections, and includes

- Purpose and effects of the drug (clinical pharmacology)
- Indications for the drug
- Contraindications (conditions under which the drug should not be given)
- Adverse reactions to the drug
- Precautions that should be noted
- Warnings concerning the use of the drug
- Drug abuse and dependence information
- Overdosage information related to the drug
- Dosage and administration information
- The drug form—tablet, liquid, etc.

Pregnancy risk category is in "precautions" section. Table 19-6 (see on student resources website) shows pregnancy risk categories.

STORAGE OF DRUGS

Medical assistants must be attentive to storage conditions of drugs. Generally, medications should not be exposed to

- Sunlight
- Bright light
- Moisture
- Extremes in temperature

Key Focus: Medical assistants should advise clients to store medications in a cool, dry place, and to ensure that containers are always kept airtight. The bathroom and kitchen should be avoided as storage areas because of excessive humidity and warmth.

Pharmacology

Some drugs are particularly sensitive and will rapidly deteriorate or become ineffective if subjected to these conditions. The standard storage instructions for labeling pharmacotherapeutic agents in the United States are as follows:

- Store below −18°C
- Store below −5°C
- Store at 2–8°C
- Store below 8°C
- Store below 25°C
- Store below 30°C

Key Focus: The temperature conditions of various drugs are often critical. Many drugs, especially those of a biological origin, need to be stored between 0°C and 4°C. Common examples are insulin and vaccine preparations.

Attention is given to issues surrounding the correct storage of drugs so that they maintain their effectiveness. Table 19-7 (see on student resources website) shows the suggested time intervals for various preparations.

Visit www.pearsonhighered.com/healthprofessionsresources to access figures and tables available on the student resources website. Click on view all resources and select Medical Assisting from the choice of disciplines. Find this book and you can see all respective tables and figures.

Pharmacology

CHAPTER 20
Drug Calculations

To prevent medication errors, medical assistants must master adding, subtracting, multiplying, and dividing whole numbers, fractions, and decimals. They must calculate dosages of drugs by weight and measures of volume.

MEASUREMENT SYSTEMS

- Metric system (most commonly used)
- Apothecary system (the oldest system, which is rarely used)
- Household system (used in patient education)

These systems have three basic units of measurement:

- Weight: milligrams, grams, and grains
- Volume: milliliters and ounces
- Length: inches, millimeters, and centimeters

The Metric System and the International System

The metric system is the most popular system used today for drug prescriptions and administration.

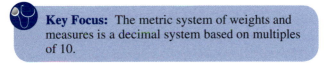

Key Focus: The metric system of weights and measures is a decimal system based on multiples of 10.

Drug Calculations

Three basic units of measurement:

1. Length—1 meter (m) = 39.37 inches. Table 20-1 shows the metric units of length.
2. Volume—1 liter (L) = 1,000 mL = 1,000 cubic centimeters (cc). Table 20-2 shows metric units of volume.
3. Weight—1 gram (g) = the volume of 1 mL in cc. Table 20-3 shows metric units of weight.

Table 20-1 *Metric Units of Length*

1 meter =	10 decimeters (dm)
	100 centimeters (cm)
	1,000 millimeters (mm)
1,000 meters =	1 kilometer (km)

Table 20-2 *Metric Units of Volume*

1 liter =	10 deciliters (dL)
	100 centiliters (cL)
	1,000 milliliters (mL)

Table 20-3 *Metric Units of Weight*

1 gram =	10 decigrams (dg)
	100 centigrams (cg)
	1,000 milligrams (mg)
1 milligram =	1,000 micrograms (mcg)
1 kilogram =	1,000 grams (g)

Five common prefixes are used to indicate units of measure:

micro	=	one millionth	=	μ (as in "μL")
milli	=	one thousandth	=	m (as in "mL")
centi	=	one hundredth	=	c (as in "cm")
deci	=	one tenth	=	d (as in "dL")
kilo	=	one thousand	=	k (as in "kg")

Table 20-4 presents the common metric equivalents.

The Apothecary System

The apothecary system is the oldest system used for the measurement of volume. Table 20-5 shows the apothecary units of volume.

The apothecary abbreviation always goes before the quantity.

$$gr \; \bar{x} = grains \; 10$$

Table 20-4 *Commonly Used Metric Equivalents*

Weight Measures	Volume Measures
1 milligram (mg) = 0.001 gram (g) or 1,000 micrograms (μg)	1 milliliter (mL) or 1 cubic centimeter (cc) = 0.001 liter (L)
1 centigram (cg) = 0.01 g	1 centiliter (cL) = 0.01 L
1 decigram (dg) = 0.1 g	1 deciliter (dL) = 0.1 L
1,000 mg or 0.001 kilogram (kg) = 1 g	1,000 mL = 1 L
1 dekagram (dag) = 10 g	1 dekaliter (daL) = 10 L
1 hectogram (hg) = 100 g	1 hectoliter (hL) = 100 L
1 kg = 1,000 g	1 kiloliter (kL) = 1,000 L

Table 20-5 *Apothecary Units of Volume*

Unit	Volume	Symbol
Minim	1 drop of water	♏ or min
Fluidram	60 minims	f℈
Fluidounce	8 fluidrams	f℥
Pint	16 fluidounces	pt
Quart	2 pints	qt
Gallon	4 quarts	gal

Table 20-6 shows the apothecary units of weight.

Key Focus: The apothecary system is rarely used, and only for a few drugs: nitroglycerin, aspirin, codeine, phenobarbital, and phenergan with codeine.

Table 20-6 *Apothecary Units of Weight*

Unit	Weight	Symbol
Grain	Basic unit	Gr
Scruple	20 grains	℈
Dram	60 grains	℥
Ounce	8 drams	℥ or oz
Pound	12 ounces	lb

Table 20-7 *Common Roman Numerals and Their Arabic Equivalents*

Roman Numerals	Arabic Equivalents	Roman Numerals	Arabic Equivalents
I	1	XVI	16
II	2	XVII	17
III	3	XVIII	18
IV	4	XIX	19
V	5	XX	20
VI	6	XXI	21
VII	7	XXII	22
VIII	8	XXIII	23
IX	9	XXIV	24
X	10	XXV	25
XI	11	XXVI	26
XII	12	XXVII	27
XIII	13	XXVIII	28
XIV	14	XXIX	29
XV	15	XXX	30

When interpreting a drug order or reading a drug label, it is helpful to know the common Roman numerals and their Arabic equivalents (see Table 20-7).

Key Focus: The Arabic numbers 1 to 30 are often used in allied health. Students should be familiar with larger Roman numerals: L (50), C (100), D (500), M (1,000).

Table 20-8 *Common Household Abbreviations*

Unit	Abbreviation	Equivalents
Drop	gtt	60 drops = 1 tsp
Teaspoon	t (or tsp)	6 tsp = 1 oz
Tablespoon	T (or tbsp)	1 T = 3 t
ounce (fluid)	oz (or fl)	2 T = 1 oz
ounce (weight)	oz	1 pound (lb) = 16 oz
Cup	cup	1 cup = 8 oz
Pint	pt	1 pt = 2 cups
Quart	qt	1 qt = 4 cups = 2 pt
Gallon	gal	4 qt = 1 gal

Household System

Household measurements are calculated by using common home containers. The only household units of measurement used for medications are units of volume. Table 20-8 shows common household equivalents.

Key Focus: Household system measurements should not be used for dosages. They are not consistent enough for medication measurements.

Conversions Between Measurement Systems

Medications are usually given in grams or grains. Often, what is available is different, either in units or in the system. To convert between systems easily, memorize the equivalents provided in Tables 20-9 and 20-10.

Table 20-9 *Volume Equivalents*

Metric System	Apothecary System	Household Measurements
–	1 minim	1 drop
1 milliliter	15–16 minims	15–16 drops
5 milliliters	1 dram (60 minims)	1 teaspoon (60 drops)
15 milliliters	4 drams (3 teaspoons)	1 tablespoon
30 milliliters	1 ounce (8 drams)	2 tablespoons (1 ounce)
180 milliliters	6 ounces	1 teacup
240 milliliters	8 ounces	1 glass or 1 cup
473 milliliters	1 pint	1 pint (16 ounces)
946 milliliters (1 liter)	1 quart	1 quart (32 ounces) (2 pints)
3,784 milliliters	4 quarts	1 gallon

Drug Calculations

Length Measurements

The metric and English household equivalents for length are rarely used for drug dosage calculations, but you should be able to convert between them in the medical clinic for the following types of measurements:

- Height
- Head circumference of infants
- Abdominal girth
- Wound size

Table 20-10 *Weight Equivalents*

Metric System	Apothecary System	Household Measurements
0.60 milligrams (mg)	gr 1/100	–
0.5 milligrams (mg)	gr 1/120	–
0.4 milligrams (mg)	gr 1/150	–
0.3 milligrams (mg)	gr 1/200	–
0.2 milligrams (mg)	gr 1/300	–
1,000 micrograms	gr 1/60	–
4 mg	gr 1/15	–
6 mg	gr 1/10	–
10 mg	gr 1/6	–
15 mg	gr ¼	–
60 mg	1 grain	–
1 gram (1,000 mg)	15 grains	–
5 grams	1 dram	–
15 grams	4 drams	–
30 grams	8 drams	1 ounce
454 grams	12 ounces	1 pound
1 kg (1,000 grams)	–	2.2 pounds

Table 20-11 shows linear equivalents for metric and household systems.

BASIC MATH

Fractions, ratios, percentages, and decimals are important. For example, 1/2 is the same as 0.5 and the ratio of 1:2.

Table 20-11 *Linear Equivalents for the Metric and Household Systems*

Metric	Household
2.5 centimeters or 25 millimeters	1 inch
30 centimeters	12 inches (1 foot)
1 meter	39.4 inches

To compare an ordered drug amount to an amount on hand, ratios are often used. For percentages in fractions, divide the numerator (top number) by the denominator (bottom number). The decimal point is moved two spaces to the right, creating a percentage.

Example:

$$\frac{1}{2} = 1 \div 2 = 0.50$$
$$0.50 = 50.0 = 50\%$$

A proportion involves the comparison of two ratios. It results from a fraction. For the fraction 1/2, the proportion could be 10/20 = 1/2, or 10:20::1:2. Table 20-12 shows examples of mathematical equivalents.

Key Focus: Medication errors are of the utmost importance to avoid. Drug dosage calculation is one of the factors that may commonly cause medication errors. You should always calculate carefully, checking your measurements and calculations with a coworker.

Table 20-12 *Mathematical Equivalents*

Fractions	Ratios	Percentages	Decimals
1/1,000	1:1,000	0.1	0.001
1/200	1:200	0.5	0.005
1/100	1:100	1	0.01
1/4	1:4	25	0.25
1/2	1:2	50	0.50
2/3	2:3	66	0.66
3/4	3:4	75	0.75
7/8	7:8	88	0.88

DRUG DOSAGE CALCULATIONS

Medications may be prepared in solid forms, oral liquids, or injectable solutions calculated with the formula method.

Formula Method

$$\frac{D \text{ (desired amount)}}{H \text{ (dose on hand)}} \times Q \text{ (quantity)} = X \text{ (amount to be given)}$$

$$\frac{D}{H} \times Q = X$$

Example 1:

A physician ordered:	10 mg diazepam, 1 tablet at bedtime (desired amount)
On hand:	5 mg tablets (quantity)

How many tablets should the patient receive?

$$\frac{10 \text{ mg}}{5 \text{ mg}} \times 1 \text{ tablet} = \frac{10}{5} = 2 \text{ tablets}$$

Example 2:

A physician ordered: Diabinese 150 mg p.o. b.i.d.
On hand: Diabinese 100 mg tablets
   How many tablets should the patient receive?

Ordered: 150 mg
On hand: 0.1g = 0.100 = 100 mg/tab

$$\frac{150 \text{mg}}{10 \text{mg}} \times 1 \text{ tablet} = 1\frac{1}{2} \text{tablets}$$

Key Focus: When calculating dosages for medications in solid form, the drug amount is determined per tablet or capsule. When the drug is in a liquid form, the medication (e.g., mg, mEq, mcg) is dissolved in the solution (e.g., mL, oz).

Pediatric Dosage Calculations

It is imperative that the calculations be exact when administering medications to a child.

Fried's Rule

This rule is used for children younger than 1 year of age and is based on the age of the child in months.

$$\frac{\text{Age of child in months}}{150 \text{ pounds (average adult weight)}} \times \text{Average adult dose}$$

$$= \text{Child's dose}$$

Clark's Rule

This rule is based on the weight of the child. It is more accurate than other pediatric methods.

$$\frac{\text{Weight of child in pounds}}{150 \text{ pounds (average adult weight)}} \times \text{Adult dose}$$

$$= \text{Child's dose}$$

Young's Rule

This rule is used for children older than 1 year of age.

$$\frac{\text{Child's age years}}{\text{Child's age in years} + 12} \times \text{Adult dose} = \text{Child's dose}$$

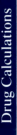

Key Focus: There are pediatric drug books available for use in administering correct dosages to children.

Chapter 21
Administering Medications

Drug administration is one of the most important tasks for a medical assistant. Its principles include

- Medication administration routes
- Dosage calculations
- Parenteral injection techniques
- Ten rights of drug administration
- Educating the patient

TEN RIGHTS OF DRUG ADMINISTRATION

Before administering any medication, medical assistants must look at the 10 "rights" of drug administration:

- Right patient
- Right drug
- Right dose
- Right time
- Right route
- Right documentation
- Right client education
- Right to refuse
- Right assessment
- Right evaluation

Preparation of Drug Administration

The medical assistant should understand uses, interactions, contraindications, and adverse effects of many common drugs, especially those often prescribed in their medical facility. Patients need medical assistants to explain many aspects of drugs that are prescribed to them.

- Medical assistants often interview patients
- They must be aware of changes in patient's condition that could affect drug therapy, and alert the physician

Drug Allergies

The physician must be aware of all medications being taken by a patient before prescribing. All types of medications have the potential to interact negatively. The medical assistant must maintain a complete, accurate patient medication list in the patient's chart, updating it during every patient appointment. It is important to

- Ask the patient about any drug allergies, as well as any new drugs being taken, during every visit
- If applicable, document in the patient chart "no known drug allergies" or "NKDA"

Site of Administration

Always check the site of administration before administering a drug. For oral medications, the patient must be able to swallow normally, and not be nauseous. Some oral drugs should not be given if the patient has had anything to eat or drink. For injectable drugs, the skin should be checked for problem areas, including

- Moles, birthmarks, or warts
- Scars, traumatic injuries, or tattoos
- Redness, rash, or burns
- Edema, cyanosis, or paralyzed areas
- Site of a mastectomy

The medical assistant should inform the physician if he or she is unsure of any of these conditions.

Patient Consent Form

Many physicians require the signing of a patient consent form before giving an injection, such as for vaccines. The form provides information about the medication or vaccine, and lists possible adverse or side effects. The patient must sign the form after having any questions answered, prior to the injection being given.

GUIDELINES FOR DRUG ADMINISTRATION

- Assemble the equipment.
- Follow standard precautions.
- Check for drug allergies.
- Check the medication order.
- Check label on drug container three times.
- Check the expiration date on the drug label; use only if date is current.
- Recheck calculation of drug dose with another medical assistant, nurse, or physician.
- Pour tablets or capsules in cap of container.
- Verify patient identification.
- Pour liquid at eye level. The meniscus (lower curve of liquid) should be at the line of the desired dose.
- Dilute medications that irritate gastric mucosa (potassium, aspirin) or give with meals.
- Administer only those medications that you have prepared.
- Do not prepare drugs to be administered by another person.
- Stay with patient until drug is taken.
- Give no more than 1 mL subcutaneously.
- Administer no more than 2.5–3 mL of medication intramuscularly at one site.
- Infants should receive no more than 1 mL of solution intramuscularly at one site.

- Never recap needles.
- Discard needles and syringes into appropriate containers.
- Discard unused solutions from ampoules.
- Keep narcotics in a double-locked drawer or closet.

ROUTE OF ADMINISTRATION

The route of administration should be indicated when the drug is ordered.

Oral Drug Administration

- The drug is taken by mouth and swallowed by the patient.
- Solid medications should be taken with enough water to move them to the stomach.
- Liquid medications are ideal for children.
- Solid drugs should not be given to children until they can safely swallow them.
- Oral syringes are an ideal way to give liquid medications to children.

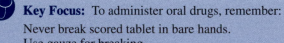

Key Focus: To administer oral drugs, remember:
Never break scored tablet in bare hands.
Use gauze for breaking.
Never crush enteric tablets.
Never open time-release capsules.
Keep drugs from children.

Buccal Administration

The term "buccal" pertains to the inside of the cheek.

- The medication must be placed between the cheek and gum.

Administering Medications

- Be sure that medication is not swallowed by patient.
- No food or water is permitted until the medication is completely absorbed.

Sublingual Administration

The medication is placed under the tongue until it dissolves (e.g., nitroglycerin for anginal pain).

Topical Drug Forms

Topical medications can be applied to the skin:
- Creams and ointments
- Gels
- Lotions
- Skin patches

or mucosal membranes:
- Eyedrops, eardrops, and nose drops
- Eye ointments
- Vaginal creams
- Rectal and vaginal suppositories
- Sterile douche solutions
- Sublingual or buccal tablets

Transdermal Drug Delivery (TDD)

Transdermal medication is stored in a patch and absorbed through the skin, for systemic effect. It is mostly used for administration of nitroglycerin, contraceptives, nicotine, scopolamine, insulin, drugs used to treat allergic reactions.

- Change patches on a regular basis.
- Rotate the site of patches.
- Before applying a transdermal patch, verify that the previous patch has been removed.

Instillations

Instillations are liquid medications usually given as drops, ointments, or sprays (eyedrops, eye ointments, eardrops, nose drops, nasal sprays). Ophthalmic, otic, and nasal drug administrations are used to treat local conditions.

> **Key Focus:** Eardrops should be administered when the medication is at room temperature. For children, pull down and back on the auricle of their ear. After 3 years of age, administration is accomplished in the same manner as for adults (pulling up and back on the auricle).

Suppositories

Medications administered as suppositories are given for local and systemic absorption.

- Rectal suppositories
  - Patient should remain on his or her side for 20 minutes after insertion.
  - They melt and are absorbed at body temperature.
- Vaginal suppositories
  - They are generally inserted into the vagina using an applicator.
  - Patient should be in the lithotomy position.

Administration of Inhalation Medications

Inhalation therapies are supplied in the form of

- Sprays
- Powders
- Water vapor
- Gases (oxygen, carbon dioxide, and nitrous oxide)

Inhalers are used for dispensing oral medications into the respiratory tract. The equipment used for this route is the metered inhaler (nebulizer).

Key Focus: Patients may use a metered-dose inhaler (MDI) at home. The medical assistant must ensure that the patient is trained in the correct use of the MDI.

Medications utilized via an MDI include

- Bronchodilators
- Mucolytic agents
- Steroids

Parenteral Medication Administration

Administering a medication through injection is referred to as parenteral administration. This is the most efficient method of drug administration but can also be the most hazardous.

Key Focus: It is vital to decrease or eliminate needlestick injuries and transfer of bloodborne diseases, such as hepatitis and human immunodeficiency virus (HIV).

Equipment Used for Parenteral Injections

Needles: A needle consists of the hub, hilt, shaft, and point (see Figure 21-1). There are two types: disposable and nondisposable. *Gauge* refers to diameter of the needle lumen (circular, hollow space inside needle). Needle gauges (G) range from 14 to 32; lengths vary from 3/8 to 1.5 inches for standard injections.

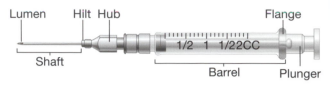

Figure 21-1 *Hypodermic needle.*

A larger gauge indicates a smaller diameter of the needle lumen. For example, a 16-gauge needle is much larger than a 30-gauge needle. Table 21-1 shows gauge and length of needles for different types of injections.

Syringes: These are classified as disposable or nondisposable. All syringes consist of the following:

- Plunger
- Barrel
- Flange
- Tip

Table 21-1 *Needle Gauges for Different Types of Injections*

Type of Injection	Needle Gauge	Length of Needle (inches)
Intradermal	27–28	3/8 to 1/2
Subcutaneous	25–26	1/2 to 5/8
Intramuscular	18–23	1 to 3
Intravenous lines	18–22	1 to 1.5
Trauma care	14–18 (the largest)	Longer than 1 inch depending on usage

There are a variety of syringes, including

- Hypodermic
- Insulin
- Tuberculin
- Prefilled

Ampoules: An ampoule is a small, sealed glass flask, usually holding a single dose of medication. The top of the ampoule is broken off, and the solution is aspirated into the syringe.

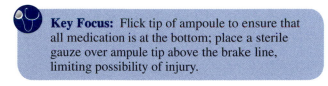

Key Focus: Flick tip of ampoule to ensure that all medication is at the bottom; place a sterile gauze over ampule tip above the brake line, limiting possibility of injury.

Vials: A vial is a small glass or plastic container with a rubber stopper, intended to hold medicine.

Prefilled cartridge injection systems: Prefilled syringes contain a premeasured amount of medication in a disposable, sterile cartridge with a needle attached. Most of these systems offer

- Reusable, plastic full-length holders designed for stability during injections
- Easy disposal of the cartridge after use
- A wide range of medications, including narcotics and intravenous flush products
- Tamper-evident packaging
- A wide variety of fill sizes

Intradermal Injections
- A small amount of medication is injected to form a wheal.

- Preferred areas for intradermal injections include the ventral mid-forearm, the chest area, and the upper back (the chosen site should be free of hair).
- This technique is commonly used for allergy skin testing or tuberculin tests.
- The amount of medication injected ranges from 0.01 to 0.1 mL.
- Absorption rate is slow.
- Equipment includes needle with a gauge of 25 to 27, a length of 3/8 to 1/2 inch, and a syringe with 1 mL calibrated in 0.01-mL increments.
- Insert the needle, and bevel up at a 10° to 15° angle (see Figure 21-2).
- Slowly inject the medication to form a small wheal or bleb (small raised area).
- The injection site should NOT be massaged following the injection.

> **Key Focus:** Patients must be told to call their healthcare provider or M.A. if developing a rash, itching, hives, or elevated temperature from administration of a drug.

Subcutaneous Injections

- Prepare the medication in a 1- to 3-mL syringe.
- Give these injections into the layer of fatty tissue that lies below the skin. You should pinch the injection site before injecting certain medications (such as insulin).
- Sites for subcutaneous injections include the abdomen, the upper lateral part of the arm, the anterior thigh, and the upper ventrodorsal gluteal areas.
- The gauges range from 25 to 26, using a 1/2-inch to 5/8-inch needle. For heparin or insulin, the recommended needle is also 3/8 inch and 25–26 gauges.

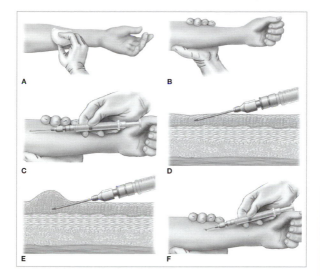

Figure 21-2 *Intradermal skin test.*

- The needle should be inserted at a 45° angle to the skin for average-weight patients, and for obese patients the angle may be 90° (see Figure 21-3).
- Check the previous rotation sites and select a new area for injection (see Figure 21-4).
- The injection sites should be altered accordingly if repeated doses are necessary.

Key Focus: With subcutaneous heparin, do not aspirate. This may damage surrounding tissues, causing bleeding or bruising, due to heparin's anticoagulant properties.

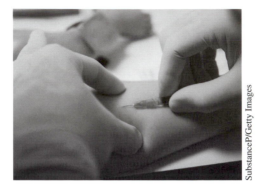

Figure 21-3 *Subcutaneous injection needle position.*

SubstanceP/Getty Images

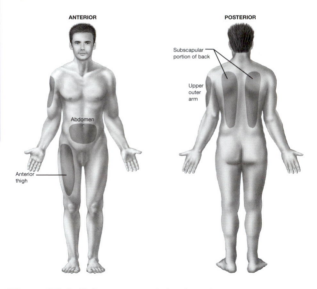

ANTERIOR

POSTERIOR

Subscapular portion of back

Upper outer arm

Abdomen

Anterior thigh

Figure 21-4 *Subcutaneous injection sites.*

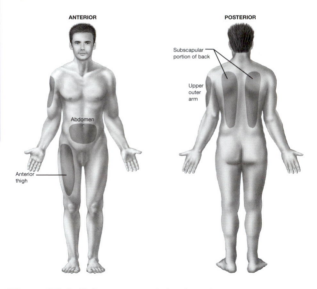
Administering Medications

Intramuscular Injections

- Intramuscular injections are given into the muscles when
  - Drugs will irritate the subcutaneous tissues
  - A more rapid absorption is desired
  - The volume of the medication to be injected is large
- The angle of insertion is 90°; preferred sites are the gluteus medius, vastus lateralis, deltoid, and ventrogluteal muscles of the adult, and the vastus lateralis of the infant and child (see Figure 21-5).
- Recommended gauge when injecting into the deltoid muscle is 23 to 25, with a 5/8-inch to 1-inch needle.
- Deltoid and tricep muscles receive no more than 1 mL; gluteus minimus 3–5 mL; vastus lateralis 1–2 mL.

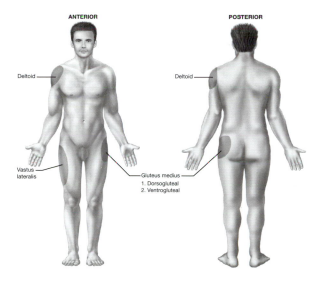

Figure 21-5 *Intramuscular injection sites.*

- For the vastus lateralis and gluteus muscles, the needle gauge should be between 18 and 23, with needle length ranging from 1 to 1½ inches.
- Inject the medication slowly and with smooth, even pressure on the plunger.
- The middle third of the muscle of the vastus lateralis is the site for intramuscular injections.

Key Focus: The reason for aspirating before intramuscular injection is to ensure that the needle is not in a blood vessel. If blood appears in the syringe, withdraw the needle, discard the syringe, and prepare a new injection.

Z-Track Method

Some intramuscular drugs irritate the skin and subcutaneous tissues. Therefore, leakage must be prevented from the deep muscle back into the upper subcutaneous layers (e.g., when injecting ferrous oxide).

- The Z-track technique displaces the upper tissue laterally before the needle is inserted. See Figure 21-6.
- The dorsogluteal, ventrogluteal, and vastus lateralis muscles are the best sites for the Z-track method. Never use the deltoid muscle for this technique.
- When you draw up a prescribed medication into the syringe, add 0.3 to 0.5 mL of air to the syringe.
- Air injection clears the needle, prevents medication from leaking into subcutaneous tissue after injection.
- Attach a new 2-inch sterile needle to syringe—prevents introducing medication that could irritate tissue.
- Wait several seconds after injecting the medication before you withdraw the needle.

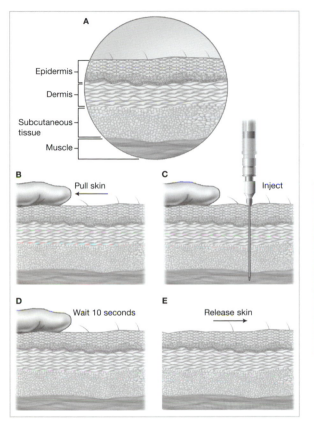

A

Epidermis

Dermis

Subcutaneous
tissue

Muscle

B
Pull skin

C
Inject

D
Wait 10 seconds

E
Release skin

Figure 21-6 *Z-track method.*

- Do not massage the area.
- Observe patient for at least 15 minutes for adverse reactions (not untoward reactions).

Pediatric Injection Sites

Infants and children have less muscle development than adults. Intramuscular injections are usually given in the vastus lateralis and ventrogluteal sites. The vastus lateralis is large and thick. The deltoid muscle is not developed and should be avoided. The dorsogluteal region is not used in younger children, to avoid hitting the sciatic nerve.

- For a child who has been walking for about 1 year—use the ventrogluteal or dorsogluteal site
- Adult injection sites can be used for older, well-developed children
- For a child who needs to be restrained, the vastus lateralis site may be easier to use
- Vaccines are the most common injections given to children; they are given IM, usually using a 25-gauge, 5/8-inch needle; this is based on size of child; the shortest needle that will reach the muscle should be used

  - If two or more vaccines must be given into same area, injections must be at least 1-inch apart
  - The specific location of each vaccine must be documented

Intravenous Therapy

Intravenous therapy is a process that involves administering fluids and solutions directly into a patient's vein.

To calculate intravenous flow rates, the formula method is used. Rate is calculated in drops per minute (gtt/min):

$$V(\text{volume in mL}) \div T(\text{time in minutes})$$
$$\times C(\text{drop factor in gtt/mL}) = R(\text{rate})$$

Key Focus: Patients should be advised to contact their physician if complications are experienced from the administration of any medications. Complications may include redness, swelling, or pain at an intravenous site, and swelling of the legs, feet, or both.

The following equipment and supplies for preparing an intravenous tray are required:

- Absorbent disposable sheet
- Alcohol prep pads
- Betadine swabs
- Disposable tourniquet
- Intravenous setup
- Intravenous tubing with attached filter
- Intravenous catheter
- Bag of intravenous fluid labeled with type
- Syringe
- Port cap
- Disposable gloves
- Gauze (2 × 2)
- Intravenous setup tray
- Intravenous pole with pump

Key Focus: State laws mandate whether medical assistants can be licensed to start intravenous infusions. In many states where they are certified and have had advanced training, they may prepare the intravenous tray for administration of the intravenous fluids.

ADMINISTERING VACCINES

Medical assistants are allowed to administer various vaccines in most states.

- A vaccination is the process of giving an injection or other form of antibody to protect an individual from an infectious disease.
- Vaccines are classified as live attenuated and inactivated.
- Live attenuated vaccines are produced from viruses or bacteria in a laboratory.
  - Polio (Sabin and oral) (the injectable Salk vaccine is used in some European countries, not in the United States)
  - Measles/mumps/rubella (MMR)
  - Yellow fever
  - Varicella zoster (human herpes virus 3)
  - BCG (bacillus of Calmette and Guérin) (for tuberculosis)
- Inactivated vaccines can be composed of whole viruses, bacteria, or fractions of either. Examples include
  - Polio (Salk)
  - Rabies
  - Influenza
  - Hepatitis A
  - Typhus
  - Pertussis
  - Typhoid
  - Cholera

Toxoids

Toxoids are inactivated toxins used to protect against disease caused by toxins produced by the invading bacterium. They are prepared by treating the toxins to destroy the toxic part of the molecules while retaining the antigenic parts. Diphtheria and tetanus vaccines are toxoids.

Recombinant Vaccines

- Subunit vaccine produced by a genetically engineered microorganism
- Example: vaccine against the hepatitis B virus

Conjugate Vaccines

Conjugate vaccines represent an important alternative over purified polysaccharide vaccines because they are effective in young children.

Recommended vaccinations and immunization schedules for both children and adults are shown in three figures on the student resources website (see Figures 21-7 through 21-9). Table 21-2 (see on the student resources website) shows some important immunizing agents for humans and their routes of administration.

> Visit www.pearsonhighered.com/healthprofessionsresources to access figures and tables available on the student resources website. Click on view all resources and select Medical Assisting from the choice of disciplines. Find this book and you can see all respective tables and figures.

APPENDICES

Appendices

APPENDIX A
Common Medical Terms and Misspelled Terms

COMMON MEDICAL TERMS

acquired immune
  deficiency syndrome
acute
adverse drug reaction
albumin
anemia
anterior
antidiuretic hormone
atherosclerosis
attention deficit
  hyperactivity disorder
blood pressure
cancer
capsule
carcinoma
cerebrovascular accident
  (stroke)
chemistry panel
chemotherapy
chief complaint
chronic obstructive
  pulmonary disease
colitis
complete blood count
coronary artery
creatinine
cubic centimeter

deep venous thrombosis
diabetes mellitus
dialysis
diarrhea
differential diagnosis
dilation and curettage
diverticulitis
do not resuscitate
dyspnea
edema
electrolyte
embolism
epilepsy
erythrocyte
fracture
globulin
glucose
gram
hematocrit
hematuria
hemoglobin
hormone
hypertension
hysterectomy
idiopathic
intensive care
international unit

Common Medical Terms

intradermal
intramuscular
in vitro
in vivo
irritable bowel syndrome
leukemia
leukocyte
ligament
medical history
milligram
myocardial infarction
normal sinus rhythm
osteoarthritis
ovaries
peptic ulcer
platelet
pneumonia
premenstrual syndrome
prolapse
proteinuria

pulmonary
radiation
rebound
renal
review of systems
rheumatoid arthritis
seizure
shortness of breath
sinusitis
sleep apnea
subcutaneous
syndrome
tablet
tendon
thyroid
unit
upper respiratory infection
urinalysis
urinary tract infection
vital signs

MISSPELLED TERMS

abscess
additive
aerosol
agglutination
albumin
anastomosis
aneurysm
anteflexion
arrhythmia
bilirubin
bronchial
calcaneus

capillary
cervical
chromosome
cirrhosis
clavicle
curettage
cyanosis
defibrillator
ecchymosis
effusion
epididymis
epistaxis

eustachian
fissure
glaucoma
gonorrhea
hemorrhage
hemorrhoids
homeostasis
humerus
idiosyncrasy
ileum
ilium
infarction
intussusception
ischemia
ischium
larynx
leukemia
malaise
malleus
mellitus
menstruation
metastasis
neuron
occlusion
oscilloscope
osseous
palliative
parasite
parenteral
parietal
paroxysmal
pemphigus
percussion

perforation
pericardium
perineum
peristalsis
peritoneum
petit mal
pharynx
pituitary
plantar
pleura
pleurisy
pneumonia
polyp
prophylaxis
prostate
prosthesis
pruritus
psoriasis
pyrexia
respiratory
roentgenology
sagittal
sciatica
serous
sphincter
sphygmomanometer
squamous
staphylococcus
suppuration
trochanter
venous
wheal
xiphoid

APPENDIX B
Proofreader's Marks

style of type

wf	Wrong font (size or style of type)
lc	lower case letter
lc	Set in LOWER CASE
c	capital letter
Caps	SET IN capitals
c+lc	Set in lower case with INITIAL CAPITALS
sc	SET IN small capitals
c+sc	SET IN SMALL CAPITALS with initial capitals
rom.	Set in roman type
ital.	Set in italic type
ital.caps	SET IN ITALIC capitals
lf	Set in lightface type
bf	Set in boldface type
bf ital.	Set in boldface italic
bf caps	Set in boldface CAPITALS
	Superior figure
	Inferior figure 2

position

⌐	Move to right
⌐	Move to left
ctr	⌐ Center ⌐
⊔	Lower (letters or words)
⌐	Raise (letters or words)
‖	Straighten type (horizontally)
‖	Align type (vertically)
tr	Transpose
tr	Transpose (order letters or of words)

spacing

ld in	Insert lead (space) between lines
⌐ ld	Take out lead
	Close up; take out space
#	Close up partly; leave some space
Eq #	Equalize space between words
#	Insert space (or more space)
space out	More space between words

insertion and deletion

the /)	Caret (insert marginal addition
ℓ	Delete (take it out)
ℐ	Delete and close up
ℓ	Correct letter or word marked
stet	Let it stand (all matter above dots)

paragraphing

¶	Begin a paragraph
No ¶	No paragraph.
Run in	Run in or run on
flush	No indention

punctuation

(Use caret in text to show point of insertion)

⊙	Insert period
⋏	Insert comma
⊙	Insert colon
;/	Insert semicolon
∜/∜	Insert quotation marks
∜/∜	Insert single quotes
∜	Insert apostrophe
(set)?	Insert question mark
!	Insert exclamation point
=	Insert hyphen
1/M	Insert one-em dash
(/)	Insert parentheses
[/]	Insert brackets

miscellaneous

⊗	Replace broken or imperfect type
↺	Reverse (upside down type)
sp	Spell out (twenty 20)
au/?	Query to author
Ed/?	Query to editor
⌐	Mark off or break; start new line

APPENDIX C
Rules for Alphabetic Filing

Rules	Example
Names are filed: last name, first name, middle name, or middle initial. Each letter in the name is a separate unit	Krause, Marvin K. is placed before Krause, Marvin L.
Initials come before a full name	Brown, H. is placed before Brown, Henry
Hyphenated names are treated as one unit. This applies to the names of individuals and businesses	Amy Freeman-Smith is indexed under F for Freeman. It is considered Freemansmith for indexing purposes
Titles and initials are disregarded for filing, but placed in parentheses after the name	Dr. Beth Ann Williams is indexed as Williams, Beth Ann (Dr)
Married women are indexed using their legal name. Their husband's name can be used for cross-referencing	Mrs. Mary Jane Smith is indexed as Smith, Mary Jane (Mrs. John)
Seniority units such as Jr. and Sr. are filed in a numerical order, from first to last	Jacob James Jurgens, Sr. comes before Jacob James Jurgens, Jr.

(continued)

Alphabetic Filing

Rules	Example
Numeric seniority terms are filed before alphabetic terms	Jurgens, Jacob James III is indexed before Jurgens, Jacob James, Jr.
Mac and Mc can be filed either alphabetically as they occur or grouped together, depending on the preference of the office	
Foreign language names are indexed as one unit	Mary St. Claire is indexed as Stclaire, Mary. Carol van Damm is indexed as Vandamm, Carol
If company names are identical, the address (by state, then city, and then street) may be used in the index. The ZIP code is not used to index files	ABC Drugs, 123 Michigan Blvd., Chicago, IL is indexed before ABC Drugs, 1450 N. Ash, Kalispell, MT
If individuals' names are identical, use their birth date or their mother's maiden name. Avoid using addresses since these can change	Mark Richard Jones is indexed as Jones, Mark Richard (5/12/65) and Jones, Mark Richard (2/12/89)
Disregard apostrophes	Megan O'Connor is indexed as Oconnor, Megan
Business organizations are indexed as they are written	Lincoln Memorial Hospital is correct

Rules	Example
Disregard short terms, such as *a*, *and*, *the*, and *of*	23rd Avenue Clinic would be indexed before the Nineteenth Street Medical Center. A separate file is set up for all numeric files
Names with religious titles, such as Sister Mary Murphy, would be filed with the last name first and then with the religious title	Murphy, Sister Mary
Compound words are filed as they are written	South West Physician Service is filed before Southwest Physician Service

APPENDIX D
MyPlate Dietary Guidelines

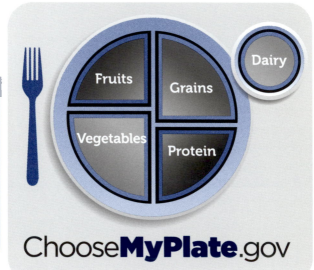

Dietary Guidelines

Today, about half of all American adults have one or more chronic diseases, often related to poor diet. The *2015–2020 Dietary Guidelines for Americans* emphasizes the importance of creating a healthy eating pattern to maintain health and reduce the risk of disease. Everything we eat and drink—the food and beverage choices we make day to day and over our lifetime—matters.

MyPlate offers messages, resources, and tools to help you make the choices that are right for you.

- **Make half your plate fruits and vegetables: Focus on whole fruits**
  - Choose whole fruits—fresh, frozen, dried, or canned in 100% juice.
  - Enjoy fruit with meals, as snacks, or as a dessert.
- **Vary your veggies**
  - Try adding fresh, frozen, or canned vegetables to salads, sides, and main dishes.
  - Choose a variety of colorful veggies prepared in healthful ways: steamed, sautéed, roasted, or raw.
- **Make half your grains whole grains**
  - Look for whole grains listed first or second on the ingredients list—try oatmeal, popcorn, whole-grain bread, and brown rice.
  - Limit grain desserts and snacks, such as cakes, cookies, and pastries.
- **Move to low-fat or fat-free milk or yogurt**
  - Choose fat-free milk, yogurt, and soy beverages (soy milk) to cut back on saturated fat.
  - Replace sour cream, cream, and regular cheese with low-fat yogurt, milk, and cheese.
- **Vary your protein routine**
  - Mix up your protein foods to include seafood, beans and peas, unsalted nuts and seeds, soy products, eggs, and lean meats and poultry.
  - Try main dishes made with beans and seafood, such as tuna salad or bean chili.
- **Drink and eat less sodium, saturated fat, and added sugars**
  - Use the Nutrition Facts label and ingredients list to limit items high in sodium, saturated fat, and added sugars.

- Choose vegetable oils instead of butter, and oil-based sauces and dips instead of ones with butter, cream, or cheese.
- Drink water instead of sugary drinks.

Source: https://choosemyplate-prod.azureedge.net/sites/default/files/misc/dietaryguidelines/myplatemywins.pdf

The official website of MyPlate is https://www.choosemyplate.gov

APPENDIX E
Nutrition (Vitamins and Minerals)

Fat-Soluble Vitamins	Deficiency Symptoms and Diseases
Vitamin A (retinol, carotene)	Retarded growth, susceptibility to infection, dry skin, night blindness, xerophthalmia, abnormal gastrointestinal function, dry mucous membranes, and degeneration of the spinal cord and peripheral nerves
Vitamin D (calciferol)	Rickets and osteomalacia
Vitamin E (tocotrienol, tocopherol)	Neurological symptoms, including ataxia, peripheral neuropathy, myopathy, and pigmented retinopathy
Vitamin K (phylloquinone)	Hemorrhage (extensive oral antibiotic therapy may cause vitamin K_2 deficiency)

Water-Soluble Vitamins	Deficiency Symptoms and Diseases
Vitamin B_1 (thiamine)	Loss of appetite, irritability, tiredness, nervous disorders, sleep disturbance, beriberi, loss of coordination, paralysis, and Wernicke–Korsakoff syndrome
Vitamin B_2 (riboflavin)	Impaired growth, weakness, lip sores and cracks at the corners of the mouth, cheilosis, photophobia, cataracts, anemia, and glossitis (riboflavin deficiency is believed to be the most common vitamin deficiency in the United States)
Vitamin B_3 (niacin)	Pellagra, characterized by dermatitis, diarrhea, dementia, and death; gastrointestinal and mental disturbances
Vitamin B_5 (pantothenic acid)	Fatigue, headaches, nausea, abdominal pain, numbness, tingling, muscle cramps, susceptibility to respiratory infections, and peptic ulcers
Vitamin B_6 (pyridoxine)	Anemia, neuritis, anorexia, nausea, depressed immunity, and dermatitis

Water-Soluble Vitamins	Deficiency Symptoms and Diseases
Vitamin B_9 (folic acid)	Anemia and spina bifida in fetal development
Vitamin B_{12} (cobalamin)	Pernicious anemia and neurological disorders
Vitamin C (ascorbic acid)	Scurvy, characterized by gingivitis, loose teeth, and slow healing of wounds; lowered resistance to infections, joint tenderness, dental caries, bleeding gums, delayed wound healing, bruising, hemorrhage, and anemia

Minerals	Deficiency Symptoms and Diseases
Calcium (Ca)	Rickets, osteomalacia (adult rickets), tetany, and osteoporosis
Copper (Cu)	Anemia and bone disease (copper deficiency is very rare in adults)
Fluoride (F)	Tooth decay and possible osteoporosis
Iodine (I)	Goiter, cretinism (congenital myxedema)—goiter is more common among women; a thyroid gland dysfunction can cause acquired myxedema, commonly known as hypothyroidism, in adults

Nutrition

(*continued*)

Minerals	Deficiency Symptoms and Diseases
Iron (Fe)	Iron-deficiency anemia and nutritional anemia
Magnesium (Mg)	Angina, constipation, depression, eating disorders, fibromyalgia, high blood pressure, insomnia, kidney stones, migraines, osteoporosis, and many others
Phosphorus (P)	Weight loss, anemia, anorexia, fatigue, abnormal growth, and bone demineralization
Potassium (K)	Impaired growth, hypertension, bone fragility, renal hypertrophy, bradycardia, and death
Sodium (Na)	Weakness, apathy, nausea, and muscle cramps in the extremities
Zinc (Zn)	Dwarfism, delayed growth, hypogonadism, anemia, and decreased appetite

APPENDIX F
CMA, RMA, CCMA, and NCMA Examinations

Category	Topics Covered
General (or Basic)	Medical terminology Anatomy and physiology Behavioral science; psychology Medical law and ethics
Administrative	Oral and written communication Records management Insurance and coding Computers and office machines Bookkeeping, collections, and credit Law and ethics
Clinical	Examination room techniques and procedures Laboratory techniques and procedures Pharmacology and medication administration Emergency procedures Specimen collection Diagnostic tests

Note: All of these examinations are basically the same, covering the topics listed above. The CCMA lists "Basic, Administrative, and Clinical," while the CMA and RMA exams list "General, Administrative, and Clinical." The NCMA has 13 content categories, but these cover the same basic required knowledge as the other exams.

Sources:
CMA – http://www.aama-ntl.org/cma-aama-exam 800-228-2262
RMA – https://www.americanmedtech.org 847-823-5169
CCMA – http://www.nhanow.com/certifications/
clinical-medical-assistant 800-499-9092
NCMA – https://www.ncctinc.com/certifications/ma.aspx
800-875-4404

CMA, RMA, and CCMA

Laboratory Requisition

Normal Laboratory Test Values

Laboratory Tests	Conventional Units	SI Units
Acid hemolysis	No hemolysis	No hemolysis
Alkaline phosphatase	14–100	14–100
Cell counts— erythrocytes		
Male	4.6–6.2 million/mm^3	$4.6–6.2 \times 10^{12}$/L
Female	4.2–5.4 million/mm^3	$4.2–5.4 \times 10^{12}$/L
Children (varies with age)	4.5–5.1 million/mm^3	$4.5–5.1 \times 10^{12}$/L
Leukocytes, total	4,500–11,000/mm^3	
Leukocytes, differential counts		
Myelocytes	0%	0/L
Band neutrophils	3–5%	$150–400 \times 10^6$/L
Segmented neutrophils	54–62%	$3,000–5,800 \times 10^6$/L
Lymphocytes	25–33%	$1,500–3,000 \times 10^6$/L

Laboratory Tests	Conventional Units	SI Units
Monocytes	3–7%	$300–500 \times 10^6$/L
Eosinophils	1–3%	$50–250 \times 10^6$/L
Basophils	0–1%	$15–50 \times 10^6$/L
Platelets	150,000–400,000/mm^3	$150–400 \times 10^9$/L
Reticulocytes	25,000–75,000/mm^3	$25–75 \times 10^9$/L
Coagulation tests		
Bleeding time	2.75–8.0 minutes	2.75–8.0 minutes
Coagulation time	5–15 minutes	5–15 minutes
D-dimer	<0.5 µg/mL	>0.5 mg/L
Factor VIII and other coagulation factors	50–150 of normal	0.5–1.5 of normal
Fibrin split products		<10 mg/L
Fibrinogen	<10 µg/mL	2.0–4.0 g/L
Partial thromboplastin time (PTT)	20–35 seconds	20–35 seconds
Prothrombin time (PT)	12.0–14.0 seconds	12.0–14.0 seconds

(continued)

Laboratory Tests	Conventional Units	SI Units
Coombs test		
Direct	Negative	
Indirect	Negative	
Corpuscular values of erythrocytes		
Mean corpuscular hemoglobin	26–34 pg/cell	26–34 pg/cell
Mean corpuscular volume	80–96 μm^3	80–96 fL
Mean corpuscular hemoglobin concentration (MCHC)	32–36 g/dL	320–360 g/L
Haptoglobin	20–165 mg/dL	0.20–1.65 g/L
Hematocrit		
Male	40–54 mL/dL	0.40–0.54
Female	37–47 mL/dL	0.37–0.47
Newborn	49–54 mL/dL	0.49–0.54
Children (varies with age)	35–49 mL/dL	0.35–0.49

Laboratory Tests	Conventional Units	SI Units
Hemoglobin		
Male	13.0–18.0 g/dL	8.1–11.2 mmol/L
Female	12.0–16.0 g/dL	7.4–9.9 mmol/L
Newborn	16.5–19.5 g/dL	10.2–12.1 mmol/L
Children (varies with age)	11.2–16.5 g/dL	7.0–0.2 mmol/L
Hemoglobin, fetal	<1.0% of total	<0.01 of total
Hemoglobin A1C	3–5% of total	0.03–0.05 of total
Hemoglobin A2	1.5–3.0% of total	0.015–0.03 of total
Hemoglobin, plasma	0.0–5.0 mg/dL	0.0–3.2 µmol/L
Methemoglobin	30–130 mg/dL	19–80 µmol/L
Erythrocyte sedimentation rate (ESR)		
Wintrobe		
Male	0–5 mm/h	0–5 mm/h
Female	0–55 mm/h	0–15 mm/h
Westergren		
Male	0–15 mm/h	0–15 mm/h
Female	0–20 mm/h	0–20 mm/h

APPENDIX I
Celsius and Fahrenheit Temperature Equivalents

Celsius	Fahrenheit
34.0	93.2
34.2	93.6
34.4	93.9
34.6	94.3
34.8	94.6
35.0	95.0
35.2	95.4
35.4	95.7
35.6	96.1
35.8	96.4
36.0	96.8
36.2	97.1
36.4	97.5
36.6	97.8
36.8	98.2
37.0	**98.6**
37.2	98.9
37.4	99.3
37.6	99.6
37.8	100.0

Celsius and Fahrenheit

Celsius	Fahrenheit
38.0	100.4
38.2	100.7
38.4	101.1
38.6	101.4
38.8	101.8
39.0	102.2
39.2	102.5
39.4	102.9
39.6	103.2
39.8	103.6
40.0	104.0
40.2	104.3
40.4	104.7
40.6	105.1
40.8	105.4
41.0	105.8
41.2	106.1
41.4	106.5
41.6	106.8
41.8	107.2
42.0	107.6
42.2	108.0
42.4	108.3

(*continued*)

Celsius	Fahrenheit
42.6	108.7
42.8	109.0

To convert Fahrenheit to Celsius: $(F - 32) \times (5/9) = C$

To convert Celsius to Fahrenheit: $(C) \times (9/5) + 32 = F$

Note: Values in bold indicate normal body temperatures.

Celsius and Fahrenheit

APPENDIX J
Blood Grouping

The two major blood groupings include the ABO (Landsteiner) system and the Rh system.

THE ABO SYSTEM

The four major blood groups are summarized in Table A-1: A, B, O, and AB.

Figure A-1 helps explain which blood groups may be donors or recipients. Type O is the universal donor, and AB is the universal recipient.

Table A-1 *Blood Group Identification*

Blood Group	Antigen	Antibody	Donor Types
O	No antigen	Anti-A and anti-B	O
A	Type A antigen	Anti-B	O and A
B	Type B antigen	Anti-A	O and B
AB	Type AB antigen	None	O, A, B, and AB

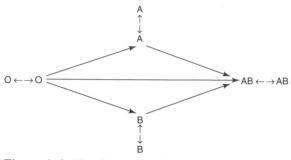

Figure A-1 *Blood donors and recipients.*

THE RH FACTOR

The Rh factor is based on an antigen first discovered on red blood cells of the Rhesus monkey. About 85% of North Americans are Rh positive and about 15% are Rh negative. The Rh factor is capable of inducing intense antigenic reactions. Table A-2 summarizes the Rh factor.

Table A-2 *The Rh Factor*

Rh Group	Rh Antigen	Donor Types
Rh positive	Yes	Only positive blood groups
Rh negative	No	Both Rh positive and Rh negative

Note: Rh incompatibility is a condition that occurs when there is a difference in the Rh blood type of pregnant women (Rh negative) and the blood type of her fetus (Rh positive). Rh immunoglobulin (RhIg) is injected into an Rh-negative pregnant woman (who has been exposed to Rh-positive antibodies due to the birth of her first child) prior to the birth of her second child.

Blood Grouping

INDEX

Note: Page numbers followed by *f* or *t* represent figures or tables respectively.